Modern Social Policy

Michael Sullivan
University of Wales, Swansea

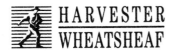

New York   London   Toronto   Sydney   Tokyo   Singapore

First published 1994 by
Harvester Wheatsheaf
Campus 400, Maylands Avenue
Hemel Hempstead
Hertfordshire, HP2 7EZ
A division of
Simon & Schuster International Group

Typeset in 10/12pt Times
by Dorwyn Ltd, Rowlands Castle, Hants

Printed and bound in Great Britain by
Biddles Ltd, Guildford and King's Lynn

British Library Cataloguing in Publication Data

A catalogue record for this book is available from
the British Library

ISBN 0–7450–1435-6 (pbk)

---

1 2 3 4 5   98 97 96 95 94

Contents

Acknowledgements

Though the responsibility for all imperfections and weaknesses in this book is, of course, mine, the help of several people in ensuring its completion demands acknowledgement.

Were it not for the encouragement and confidence of Professor W.M. Williams, my head of department for ten years until his recent retirement, my writing career would never have developed in the way that it has. In 1983, he invited me, then a relatively new member of staff, to write a book for his 'Studies in Sociology' series. That was *Sociology and Social Welfare,* to which this book is an intellectual sequel and development. More than that, he has applied his imaginative and acute intellect to all my writing projects. For his generosity in this and other matters, I acknowledge a debt of gratitude which defies words. I hope that he will accept the appearance of *Modern Social P*olicy as part payment. This, like all my work since the early 1980s, reflects an interest, shared by him, in understanding, narrating and analysing contemporary social policy.

The other constant professional source of encouragement in the last few years has been Clare Grist. She has, with deftness and tact, made suggestions that have improved this and an earlier book and has managed to keep me more or less to deadlines.

If this book draws successfully on 'real world' social policy issues and should it contribute in any way to their understanding, that is in no small part the responsibility of Susan Sullivan. While she and her colleagues in the West Wales Health Commission strive to create user-centred NHS services, and often despite government policy, I feed, parasitically on her accounts of new developments and make mental notes of how to incorporate these timely insights into my own work. I unreservedly acknowledge this debt.

Though she played no part in the development of this book, I am reminded in completing it, of my late sister-in-law, Ruth Pantoleon. She was born in the year preceding publication of the Beveridge Report. Her untimely death last year followed treatment which often represented the stretched National Health Service at its best. If ever there was need to be reminded of the fundamental importance of a welfare state and the need to fight to protect it, this sad chapter provided it.

Finally, undergraduate and postgraduate students at Swansea continue, to my surprise, to welcome the fruits of my labour. This encourages me to keep writing!

Michael Sullivan
October 1993

Introduction

This is a book about modern social policy in the United Kingdom. More particularly, it is a book about the post-war experience of welfare. Its objective is to understand the reasons why and the ways in which state social policy developed and, in the recent period, has perhaps withered. It attempts to meet this objective by outlining the social policy history of the period, by considering how competing ideas about the appropriate role of the state and social policy have interacted with and against each other, and by considering how modern social policy has unfolded in one policy area. As readers will find out, it is a story, in part, of the rise and wane of social democratic political ideas in welfare. While the social democratic settlement of 1945 commanded consensual political support, comprehensive state welfare was vouchsafed and competing ideas about social policy consigned to apparent permanent opposition. As Keynesianism faltered in the 1970s, however, things were to change and other paradigms shook the hegemony of social democratic ideas and practices. In this febrile political context, the ideas of the radical right, previously peripheral in twentieth-century British politics, found an enthusiastic promoter in the new leader of the Conservative party, Margaret Hilda Thatcher. Thatcher governments in the 1980s and the administrations headed by John Major that followed have changed dominant ideas about and practices in social policy.

These changes have prompted a number of hitherto unnecessary questions. Is the welfare state under threat? Is the British welfare system being Americanised at the time when the American system is threatening to move in the direction of the United Kingdom? Have the social policy initiatives of Conservative governments since 1979 shattered a previous consensus and built a different one? And so on. This book addresses these questions even if it sometimes provides less than definitive answers.

Readers may well recognise similarities with one of my previous books. This is especially the case in the chapters dealing with understanding social policy and understanding the state. Clare Grist of Harvester Wheatsheaf was kind enough to accept my suggestion that the earlier book should be revised. When I set about thinking about revisions, it became obvious that this book in front of you should be a sequel to rather than a revision of *Sociology and Social Welfare*. I therefore hope that readers will note differences as well as similarities and that the latter outweigh the former. The reasons for making this a new book include the obvious. Time has marched forward and there have been many developments in social policy since 1987 when *Sociology and Social Welfare* was published. At a more calculating level, the periodic reviews carried out by the Higher Education Funding Council (HEFC) in Wales and England has made many of us aware of the advantages of producing different books rather than books with different titles. More seriously, however, some of my views have changed. I take this not only as evidence of maintained suppleness of the intellectual arteries but also of the way in which Mrs Thatcher's last administration and Mr Major's two governments have exposed the intentions of Conservative social policy, even if the planned outcomes have not always followed.

This book is also less obviously sociological than its close cousin. That is not to say that I have forsaken a sociological approach. I hope that I have not. However, as readers will see if they read further, I have become convinced that the easiest way to grapple with change in post-war social policy is to chart the way in which dominant ideas and practices have been developed and superseded. As a result, the organising principles of the book have become more rooted in chronology and more conscious of party politics. In this sense, *Modern Social Policy*, is an heir to *The Politics of Social Policy* (1992) as well as of the earlier book.

The book is organised in three parts. Part I is about the context of modern social policy in the United Kingdom. The first chapter considers how social policy developed in the post-war growth economy. Put another way, it looks at how political, economic and social ideas fed into the perpetual growth of the welfare state until we became painfully aware of the fragility of the British economy in the 1970s. This chapter ends with the election, in 1979, of a Conservative government headed by a sympathiser of the radical right. Chapter 2 looks at whether and how that government, and the ones that have followed it, have changed our thinking about and our experience of welfare systems.

This contextual overture is followed, in Part II by chapters which attempt to help our understanding of the rise and fall of the old welfare state. So a chapter on understanding the modern British state is followed by two on understanding social policy. In all of the chapters in Part II there lurks an implicit, and sometimes explicit, question. That question is about how we understand the early relative success and later apparent failure of social democratic politics and reformist ideas about welfare. The final chapter in this part is devoted to looking at the unfolding of this process in one area of social policy, the provision of personal social services. The decision to present a closely argued case study was an easy one to make. It allows the reader to apply the arguments marshalled earlier in the book to a specific area of social policy. The choice of the personal social services (PSS) as the focus of this case study was a more difficult decision. In the end, the choice was made on pragmatic as well as intellectual grounds. Intellectually, it seemed a reasonable choice: the unfolding of PSS policy over the decades, its coercive and humanitarian tilts, appeared to neatly illustrate the changing fortunes of social democracy. Pragmatically, the inclusion of a PSS case study also had its attractions: particularly that it filled a gap in the literature and applied the intellectual project of the book to an area of welfare state practice. Recently, of course, this has most often been accomplished by the many books converging on the fast-moving health policy context. In my opinion, the changes in PSS have been almost as fundamental as in the National Health Service and for this reason alone a concentration on PSS policy is justified.

Part III, the final chapter of the book, returns to the difficult task of charting contemporary social policy. It considers not only the competing ideas about social policy provision and philosophy in the 1990s but also the way in which earlier influential notions have been adapted in the context of this decade. Important here, is the way in which Marshallian ideas of 'citizenship' (Marshall, 1963) have been superseded by Conservative and Labour notions of consumerism. Perhaps, this chapter muses, we are on the threshold of entirely new ways of providing and thinking about welfare.

None of this is made any easier, of course, by the political rhetoric of the major political parties. Neither admits to the demise of the welfare state and both present themselves as its protector. As we face the end of the century, however, there is a real prospect that neither the economic means nor the political will exist to exhume the spirit of Beveridge, Bevan and Butler.

PART 1

Contexts of social policy

CHAPTER 1

Social, economic and political contexts

The British Welfare State has a relatively short history and is now the subject of political debate and considerable restructuring. It was established in the 1940s with the implementation of a package of government policies that heralded state intervention on a much larger scale and in a more systematic way than ever before. A national health service (NHS) was created with the intention of providing a universal health care service free at the point of use. Compulsory secondary education, a key element of the 1944 Education Act, was introduced with the stated purpose of equalising the educational opportunities of children from different social classes. A system of social security, drawing largely on the philosophy outlined in the Beveridge Report (Beveridge, 1942), replaced the less significant social insurance schemes of the early twentieth-century Liberal governments, and was seen by many as the instrument by which poverty would be eradicated. The state replaced private charities as the main provider of personal social services, and intervened in the provision of housing in a way undreamed before the Second World War. (Useful factual summaries of the development of the welfare state can be found in Sked and Cook (1979), Marwick (1982), Morgan (1990) and Williamson (1990).)

For three post-war decades, increases in scope and momentum characterised government decisions about intervention in general and social policy intervention in particular. The foundations of the welfare state were built upon by succeeding governments. Welfare state expansion took place throughout the extended period of post-war economic growth in Britain and even in the early years of economic retrenchment. Welfare statism was seen as a reflection of a politics of consensus practised during this period by both major political parties (Marshall, 1965, pp. 180–1; 1975, p. 105; Sullivan, 1987, 1991, 1992; Hennessy, 1992; Hill, 1993).

Until the mid-1970s, large scale intervention by the state in social welfare formed part of the political orthodoxy of both major political parties. State welfare became woven into the fabric of everyday life to such an extent that Jones and Novak could claim that 'for large clusters of people . . . life from the womb to the grave is monitored by, or is dependent upon, a vast network of state social legislation and provision' (Corrigan, 1980, p. 143).

During the 1980s and the early 1990s, however, significant changes have been wrought in the way in which state welfare is delivered and in the principles underlying its provision (Johnson, 1990; Mishra, 1990). Conservative governments headed by Margaret Thatcher and her successor, John Major, have set about deconstructing what they have regarded as the cosy political consensus that underpinned the development of the post-war welfare state. The politics of conflict and competition have replaced the politics of consensus in social policy as comprehensively as they have in other areas of social and economic life (Sullivan, 1989, 1991, 1992; Taylor-Gooby, 1991). Or so it has seemed.

The introduction of internal markets within the health and personal social services (Johnson, 1990; Plant and Barry, 1991; Leathard, 1991) has presumed the growth of competition in the provision of services to replace the previous welfare state monopolies. It has also had the effect of splitting previously homogeneous welfare organisations into purchasing and providing arms (Paton, 1991; Sullivan, 1991, 1992) and of creating a quasi-private provider sector within the NHS in the form of NHS trusts. Radical changes in education have seen the advance of the self-governing school, receiving its funding direct from the Secretary of State rather than from the local education authority, and the reintroduction of academic selection of pupils at pre-secondary school age. Apparently extensive changes have occurred in the social security system, where the expansion of selectivism is credited by some as creating a British underclass (Hill, 1990) and by others as being the response to its growth (Murray, 1990; see also Dean and Taylor-Gooby, 1991; Lawson and Wilson, 1991, on this debate).

That, at least, is one interpretation of the turbulent decade of the 1980s and the early years of the 1990s. Other interpretations point to the supposed failure of new Conservative governments in this period to effect the social policy changes that were intended. They point to a gulf between reality and rhetoric, between anti-statist discourse and the creation of a strong state, to the difference between policy intention and policy outcome (O'Higgins, 1983a; Sullivan, 1984; Taylor-Gooby, 1985; Gamble, 1985, 1987). One of the objectives of this chapter is to evaluate the claim that fourteen years of Conservative government, following 1979, have led to the restructuring of ideas about welfare and the nature and ends of social policy. We will be asking whether there have been signific-ant changes in social policy direction in the last decade and a half. We will be looking at whether it is plausible to hypothesise the end of the post-war welfare state. Of course, to understand and recog-nise the destination, we have to have followed the journey. It is that journey on which we now embark. As we undertake that journey a number of questions raise themselves. What was the post-war welfare state like? On what ideas was it based? What have been the major shifts in ideas and practices in social and economic policy and what accounts for them?

This chapter is devoted to constructing a sociological history of the post-war journey from the collectivism of the Attlee admin-istration to the apparent market capitalism of the Major govern-ment. It highlights the rise and the alleged fall of welfare statism and seeks both to describe the scope of welfare state restructuring and to explain it.

Features of the post-war British state

Prelude: the war years

If most of the post-war period was characterised by large scale state intervention in civil society, then the war years themselves were forerunners of an interventionist future. The exigencies of war prompted a degree of central planning and control of industry and economy unusual in British society. The war effort was seen to require the central direction of production. A war economy se-verely curtailed the production of luxuries. Disruption of imports and of indigenous food and clothing production required the intro-duction of rationing and controls (Addison, 1982, pp. 130–1, 161–2; Morgan, 1990). The British state at war claimed to require economic sacrifices from all sections of the population. To effect such sacrifices required state intervention.

During wartime the state intervened in the control of industry in a way it had never done before. Under the Emergency Powers Act (1940), the government sought and got powers to regulate working hours and conditions, and to enforce the settlement of pay claims through a process of bipartite negotiation involving employer and employee representatives (Harris, 1984). Such was the change in levels of state intervention that one social historian has claimed that the 'direction and control of life and labour were probably more total (and more efficient) that in any other country save for Russia' (Marwick, 1974, p. 151).

The wartime coalition government also indicated its intention to intervene in the provision and control of social welfare more systematically than previous governments. The seeds of the welfare state germinated during this period.

Despite some parliamentary opposition from Conservatives, initial hostility from Prime Minister Churchill and the apparent indifference or timidity of senior Labour Ministers, the philosophy of full employment and social security enunciated in the Beveridge Report was largely accepted (Addison, 1982, pp. 223–4; Hennessy, 1992; Pimlott, 1992; Sullivan, 1992). Plans for a national health service were also developed at this time. Despite the initial lukewarm approach of the Conservative Minister, Willink, and the obstructive behaviour of the British Medical Association (BMA), the case for a national health system which was free at the point of use was made not only by the Beveridge Report but also by the evidence of semi-socialised medicine provided by the Emergency Medical Service (EMS) (Willcocks, 1967; Forsyth, 1968; Jones, 1991; see Sullivan (1992) for a full discussion of the wartime development of health policy). War also appears to have provided the final impetus for the introduction of compulsory secondary education. Though a coalition of forces had pushed for educational reform over the previous two decades, the wartime years saw the acceleration of the policy process by the President of the Board of Education and his Labour deputy (Rubinstein and Simon, 1973; Jones, 1991; Sullivan, 1992).

Consensus, for whatever reasons and however fragile, was forged around a package of interventionist policies during the war years. Whether such a consensus was one shared by all sections of

British society or merely by political leaders and senior state personnel is, of course, an open question. Elsewhere (1992) I have argued that political consensus during this period was real, though the property of the parliamentary political parties rather than of the polity. Others, including Pimlott (1988), are unprepared to go even this far. Instead, they argue that the perception of political activists at this time was of political contention rather than of agreement. A consideration of the record, however, makes it difficult to avoid the conclusion that political agreement existed, at least at the framework level of shared views about the direction of economic and social policy (Hennessy, 1992).

One thing is certain: interventionism in the war years set the scene for what was to follow.

1945–75: three decades of interventionism

State intervention in the social and economic life of British society was a constant and increasingly marked feature of the thirty years that followed Labour's landslide victory in the 1945 general election. Interventionism was accepted as an important feature in the management of the democratic socialism of the Attlee government, of Churchill's Tory democracy, of the 'age of affluence' associated with the Macmillan administrations, the technological revolution of the first two Wilson governments and the pre-Social Contract years of the early 1970s. Throughout this period Britain witnessed significant state activity in areas that had in earlier periods substantially, if not exclusively, escaped the guiding hand of state regulation and control. This more systematic intervention by the state can be illustrated by a consideration of economic and social policy between the mid-1940s and mid-1970s, to which we now turn.

Economic policy 1945–75

Despite changes of government in 1951, 1964 and 1970, continuities in economic policy can be clearly discerned during this period. These continuities seem particularly marked in three areas: the organisation and control of industry; the philosophy of economic management; and the practice of economic management.

The organisation and control of industry

In a significant speech marking the end of the Second World War on 15 August 1945, the new Labour Prime Minister – Clement Attlee – pledged his government to work for economic recovery and social justice. These goals were to be achieved through a process of transforming rather than destroying British capitalism. The organisation of industry was seen as a crucial arena for state action in the post-war transformation of British society and the British economy. Central state control of key industries was seen as essential if the government's twin aims were to be achieved. Consequently, the post-war Labour government set about creating a mixed economy where public and private enterprise coexisted alongside each other. Certain major industries were nationalised during this period: civil aviation in 1946, coal in 1947, cables and wireless and transport in 1947, electricity in 1948, gas in 1949, and steel in 1951. Although the Conservative governments of 1951–64 did not nationalise further industries, and indeed denationalised steel in 1953, little if any attempt was made to alter the balance of the mixed economy. Indeed the attitude of Conservative governments of the period to the organisation of industry may be sensed in the words of Macmillan – Prime Minister for part of the period – as creating 'a capitalism which incorporated socialism' (Barker, 1978, p. 132). Further nationalisation occurred during Labour's occupancy of government, 1964–70. British Aerospace and British Shipbuilders were brought into public ownership during this period and steel was renationalised in 1967.

The nationalisation of key industries, the creation of a mixed economy and consequent administrative changes in this period represented major state intervention in an area of the economy where it had been almost wholly absent until the 1940s. This was however simply an important, rather than an exclusive, strategy for state intervention in the organisation and control of industry during this period. Especially in the middle and latter years of this thirty-year span, other methods of direct intervention were used. By the early 1960s it had become evident that, despite public ownership and other government interventions in the economy (which are discussed later), economic growth in Britain was proceeding at a slower pace than had been hoped or than pertained in other industrial societies.

Furthermore, a process of rapid technological advancement was occurring in the developed industrial world. With the stated aim of fuelling the fires of a technological revolution in British industry, other direct interventions by the state were introduced. Again, consensus between the political parties on state intervention in the economy in this period, spanning the 1960s and the early 1970s, was evident despite differences in political emphasis.

In 1966, the then Labour government introduced the Industrial Reorganisation Corporation, which was empowered to use government capital to promote and develop industrial enterprise. It played a direct part in the modernisation and reorganisation of a number of industries including the nuclear industry, the electrical industry and the motor industry. In 1964 the same government had created a new Ministry of Technology, and its work was aided by the Industrial Expansion Act (1968), which aimed to encourage technical and scientific innovation in industry. Key aims here were the modernisation of the machine tool industry and the promotion of Britain's computer industry. The state at a central level, then, was involved in direct intervention in the control and organisation of British industry and its involvement during this later period was not limited to those public corporations which it or its predecessor Labour governments had created through nationalisation.

Although the 1970 Conservative government disbanded the Ministry of Technology and abolished the Industrial Reorganisation Corporation, it none the less reinforced state involvement and intervention in industry. It created the Department of Trade and Industry to co-ordinate commercial and industrial policies, and introduced the Industry Act (1972). The Act gave government more extensive interventionist powers in industry than it had possessed before and was supplemented by the creation of an Industrial Development Unit to implement industry policies and by an Advisory Board.

The establishment of the National Enterprise Board (NEB) by a Labour government in 1975 and the concomitant passage of yet another Industry Act permitted further extensive and direct intervention in the private sector of British industry. The NEB (a government holding company) provided extensive financial incentives to private industry in part as inducement to rationalise, modernise and reorganise.

State intervention in the organisation and control of industry in the three decades following 1945 was, then, one feature of the state's involvement in areas hitherto regulated and controlled by the market. The evidence suggests that this interventionist activity was legitimated by a party political consensus. It was, as we shall see, grounded in a philosophy of economic management shared by both major political parties.

The philosophy of economic management

Until the Second World War the state played a comparatively small role in the management of the economy. Major manufacturing industries, like minor ones, operated within a capitalist market economy where the profit motive and the price mechanism more or less successfully regulated economic exchange. The economic depression of the inter-war years took place within the context of such a market economy, as did the economic recovery of the late 1930s, albeit aided by demand for arms and by cheap raw materials and privileged credit arrangements from the colonies and Sterling Area (Harris, 1984). From 1940 (and particularly from 1945), however, the market economy principle was replaced by a philosophy of economic management that presumed and encouraged the intervention of the British state in the control and management of the economy. This new philosophy was to guide government policy and intervention into the mid-1970s and was based on the idea of demand management of the economy. Some commentators see, in this development, a major transformation of the British State (Jessop, 1980, p. 28).

In simple terms, successive governments in the period 1945–75 made attempts at macroeconomic management of the economy to maintain it at an optimum level. Governments intervened to fine tune the economy so that the twin dangers of unemployment and inflation could be avoided and steady economic growth achieved.

So the 1945 settlement included a commitment to large scale state intervention in the economy, a commitment to use state apparatuses to regulate the level of aggregate demand in the economy. A number of instruments could be and were used by governments in the post-1945 period to achieve this end. In periods where the economy was in an apparently uncontrolled upward surge, governments acted to depress the economy. So, for example, at times when production levels were rising rapidly consequent difficulties of rising inflation and shortages of labour were also likely to occur. By macro-economic intervention the state could and did act in such periods to reinstate equilibrium in the economy. Traditional features of the dampening down process included: increasing levels of taxation that would act to decrease demands for products and restrain economic activity; increases in interest rates that had the effect of restricting credit and thereby restraining investments in industry; and the consequent regulation of inflationary pressures resulting from capital inflows into the economy.

Similarly when the economy was in slump, government could and did intervene by means of state apparatus to stimulate demand. Taxation levels would be decreased to leave more money in the economy thereby encouraging consumption. Interest rates would be reduced to encourage investment in industry and to stimulate consumer expenditure. (A helpful synopsis of the mechanisms of demand management can be found in McLennan, *et al.*, 1984, pp. 93–4).

For roughly three decades this Keynesian principle of demand management of the economy apparently worked well enough. Though it did not eradicate slump/boom cycles in the economy, it certainly mitigated their effects: between 1952 and 1964 average unemployment in Britain was only 380,000 (under 1 per cent) and by 1973 it had risen to only 590,000. Discussions of the reasons for the relative success of Keynesian economic principles in practice during this period abound (see McLennan, *et al.*, 1984, pp. 94–103) as do explanations of its ultimate failure (McLennan, *et al.*, 1984, pp. 206–8). What is important here is that for about thirty years political consensus (at least between parties of government) existed. That consensus made possible, and made real, extensive state involvement in the control of the economy to maintain full employment and economic growth. The period is characterised by almost continuous interventions by state and government in economic management based on an economic philosophy unacceptable before 1940 and increasingly unpopular, in Britain and the United States at least, after 1975.

These decades of significant state involvement in the British economy were typified, then, by large scale involvement in the control and organisation of industry and an underpinning, interventionist policy of macroeconomic management. They were similarly marked by what some (Middlemas, 1979, pp. 389–429; Greenleaf, 1987) have seen as the extension of the state by means of the incorporation of both sides of industry in economic planning functions.

Economic planning and incorporation

Post-war Britain saw the creation and maintenance of a mixed economy. The state became involved in the economy at a number of levels: it took control of some industries creating a public sector of industry; it developed a framework for and agencies to assist the reorganisation of industry to keep pace with technological and other changes; it attempted to fine tune the economy to provide a context in which a modern mixed economy could flourish and provide high levels of employment. To ensure the success of a strategy for continued and controllable growth in the British economy, however, implied not only that the state should intervene in the structure of the economy and industry but also that it should intervene to incorporate British industry into the state and into the management of the economy. In free market capitalism those who owned capital and those who sold labour were competing forces. In state interventionist mixed economy Britain, attempts were made to modify that relationship so that they would be partners with each other and government in ensuring the continued prosperity of the British economy. If the continued profitability of industry and the maintenance and improvement of workers' living standards were seen as dependent, in part, on the successful intervention of the state in industry, then the limits of success were seen by successive governments as dependent on industry's ability and willingness to be part of a tripartite relationship (including industrial management and owners, trade unions and government) initiating and co-ordinating economic policy.

Governments formed by both political parties established forums for the planning and management of the economy in which tripartite involvement was of a formal or informal nature. In 1962 the Conservative government established the National Economic Development Office (NEDO). Its task was to gather information and make recommendations over a wide range of economic policy and planning. National Economic Development committees (NEDDYs) formed part of the structure of the NEDO. They consisted of economic ministers, trade unionists and industrialists.

In 1964, the newly formed Labour government established a short-lived Department of Economic Affairs (DEA). The DEA was charged with developing an indicative plan for economic growth and, unlike the Treasury with which it vied as an initiator and co-ordinator of economic policy, its deliberations consistently, if informally, included both sides of industry.

Tripartite co-operation, formal and informal, successful and unsuccessful, was initiated by governments during the 1960s and 1970s on the issues of prices and incomes and industrial relations – both seen as crucial to the management of a growth economy. The National Board for Prices and Incomes (1965) and its successors the Pay Board and the Price Commission (1972) all involved the widest representation of interests. The Commission on Industrial Relations (1969), which functioned to conciliate between employers and trade unions, had similar representation. Following the abandonment of the White Paper *In Place of Strife* in 1969, the Trades Union Congress (TUC), which had opposed the idea of legislation aimed at outlawing wild cat strikes, took on quasi-government functions of intervention in industrial disputes. During the Social Contract years (1974 on) government, employers and the TUC acted in concert (despite discordant notes and later deafening cacophony from individual trade unions) to plan for wages and prices in an economy that had become sluggish and in which unemployment was a growing and worrying problem (Robertson and Hunter, 1970, pp. 189–202).

These examples, together with the growth of quasi-autonomous non-governmental organisations such as the Manpower Services Commission – set up in 1974 to develop plans for labour market policy despite its role since 1979 as *masseur* of unemployment figures – illustrate the extension and penetration of the state in the 1960s and 1970s into previously autonomous areas and agencies of civil society. The state attempted, with some success, to incorporate previously hostile combatants as partners in the state (or quasi-state) machinery (Middlemas, 1979, pp. 430–63).

Social policy 1945–75

Following the Second World War, the activities of the state in Britain were massively increased. An interventionist state emerged to replace a liberal, largely non-interventionist, state. The interventionist state was characterised by two major features: the large scale and consistent economic intervention we have considered above, and the extension of welfare policies and creation of a welfare state which we consider now (and, in more detail, in Chapter 3).

That the state should intervene in a systematic way to provide and control welfare was, before the Second World War, a highly contentious proposition – even Keynes argued that the state should act only to provide those services which people could not provide for themselves (Marwick, 1974). However, the consensus of the war years on welfare appears to have continued into the peacetime and the welfare state was created and expanded, more or less consistently until the mid-1970s. Continuity rather than political conflict marked state involvement in welfare during this period. The apparently linear progression of welfare state expansion can be illustrated by a consideration of the social policies of the period. In this section we concentrate on three areas of provision which exemplify the points to be made: income maintenance and social security provision, education and the National Health Service. Detailed accounts of policy development and implementation in these areas exist elsewhere (e.g. Hall *et al.*, 1978; Held, 1982; McLennan, *et al.*, 1984; Johnson, 1990; Jones, 1991; Sullivan, 1991, 1992). What interests us here is the steady and apparently consensual rise of state welfare during this period.

Income maintenance and social security provision

The social security system has often been regarded as the foundation stone of the welfare state. Beveridge is, with a large degree of justice, credited as its originator and as founding father of the British welfare state. Social security provisions had existed since the early twentieth century. None the less, the scheme promoted by Beveridge (and substantially implemented by the post-war Labour government) extended and in some crucial respects transformed earlier schemes. The scheme that resulted from the National Insurance Act (1946), the National Insurance Industrial Injuries Act (1946) and the National Assistance Act (1948) was intended to provide monetary benefits to cover earnings interruptions for those insured. It was therefore to include benefits to cover periods of sickness, unemployment and maternity. It was to provide benefits to widows and orphans, the old, the industrially injured and to offer a funeral grant to rescue the poor from the perceived indignity of a pauper's grave (George, 1973, pp. 34–6; Hill, 1990). The scheme was universal in its coverage and based on the principle of insurance. Individuals contributed to the scheme while in work, and they and their families benefited from it at times of earnings interruption. Originally the scheme yielded flat rate benefits generated largely by flat rate contributions. National Assistance at a subsistence level was provided for those who for one reason or another, were ineligible, or ceased to remain eligible for National Insurance benefits.

The income maintenance and social security system did not remain unchanged over the thirty-year period under consideration. The flat rate contribution/benefit principle was abandoned in 1966 when an earnings-related unemployment benefit was introduced. This benefit was based on an earnings-related contribution and was introduced with the stated aim of acting as a cushion against frictional unemployment during a period of industrial rationalisation. New non-contributory benefits were introduced: family income supplement in 1971; a non-contributory invalidity benefit in 1974; and a child benefit scheme introduced in 1977 despite lukewarm support (Land, 1978; Hill, 1990). Other changes, reflecting the material realities of post-war Britain, also occurred. Principal among them were the relatively large numbers of claimants subsisting for long periods of time on a National Assistance/Supplementary Benefit scheme intended as a short term-safety net scheme for a small minority of claimants. None the less, continuity in social security policy was more significant than change. Both Labour and Conservative governments kept faith with the basic Beveridge principles, even in later periods when general taxation came to subsidise a greater proportion of spending in a system expanded in scope and supporting larger numbers of people (because of economic and demographic factors). As late as 1973 and 1974 Social Security Acts underwrote the Beveridge principles despite making peripheral changes and, sometimes, improvements in provision. (For a history of this period, see Kincaid, 1973; Hall *et al.*, 1978; Hill, 1990.)

Throughout this period, then, state involvement and increasing state expenditure formed the basis of maintaining and expanding, however *ad hoc* that expansion, the British income maintenance and social security system. Growth in state social expenditure rates in this area remained substantially, if not totally, unquestioned by governments formed by both major political parties. A bipartite political consensus on the place of social security in post-war British society, and on the growth of that system to respond, even if unsuccessfully, to changes in the economy, appeared to exist. That basic commitment, if not the system's administration, remained substantially unchanged until the Social Security Reviews of the mid-1980s.

Education

Continuity and growth were also the main features of state provision and policy in education during this period. That the state should intervene to provide a universal system of secondary education had been established as a bipartisan political principle in the mid-1940s. Despite seemingly significant divisions within the Labour Party in the 1950s (and between the Labour Party and the Conservative Party throughout that whole period) over the organisation of secondary schooling, the development of comprehensive education and the involvement of state agencies in setting the agenda for change was marked by a breadth of consensus. This consensus in Westminster, and possibly in British society at large, belies the apparent significance of conflict over the issue (Parkinson, 1970; Rubinstein and Simon, 1973; Fenwick, 1976; Reynolds and Sullivan, 1987; Sullivan, 1991, 1992).

The expansion of higher education, of teacher training and of further education – all bringing with them increased state expenditure and increased state involvement in planning education – was presided over by governments of both political persuasions (see Kogan, 1971, for a discussion of developments in higher education policy).

It is of course true that even during this period differences existed on where the limits of state involvement in education should be set. The Conservative governments of the period were more committed than Labour governments to the retention of a private sector in secondary education, for example (Parkinson, 1970, pp. 94–118; Sullivan, 1991).

Similarly, Labour governments were more receptive in this period to the idea of merging the misnamed private sector of higher education (universities) with the completely state controlled (albeit local state) public sector to form a unified tertiary sector of education. However, despite these differences a large measure of agreement characterised attitudes to state involvement and expenditure in education during this period.

The National Health Service

Although the National Health Service was born amidst tremendous conflict over the supposed socialisation of health (see Foot, 1975; Pimlott, 1988; Morgan, 1990 for accounts of this conflict) there existed, during the period we are presently studying, a surprising degree of political accord over its continuation. Although its creation was fiercely resisted by the Conservative opposition of the time, the 1951 Churchill government's ready acceptance of continued state intervention in health care led one of his contemporaries to quip that he had 'stolen the socialists' clothes while they were bathing'. State involvement in health was never seriously questioned by governments of this period and there was considerable agreement between the political parties over the reorganisation of the NHS in the early 1970s. Like income maintenance and education (and indeed like housing and the personal social services), the principle of state intervention and control in health appeared sacrosanct during this period.

It is interesting to note, however, that, unlike any of the other areas of provision, the NHS operated for the whole of this period with what might be termed a within-service mixed economy. That mixed economy – embracing private provision in NHS hospitals and the partial use of the price mechanism for most of the period by means of prescription, optician service and dental charges – also, interestingly, received bipartisan political support (the Labour Party in government and in practice, if not in principle, operated the mixed economy of health).

So, whereas the other areas of provision studied demonstrate a seeming consensus on state intervention and wholesale state funding, the National Health Service in operation during this period demonstrates a consensus on state intervention with mixed funding. Indeed the National Health Service in the years 1948–75 might be seen as a microcosm not only of the state's interventionist activities in welfare but also of its operation of a mixed economy.

In summarising the argument so far, then, we may conclude the following:

1. The thirty years following the Second World War were marked by a change in the nature and growth in the scope of state intervention in the social and economic life of British society.
2. This state intervention in civil society was sanctioned by succeeding governments, both Conservative and Labour and grew out of a consensus – at least at the level of political leadership – which, in effect, transformed the state.
3. The activities of this 'transformed state' were developed around the twin commitments of succeeding governments to a mixed economy and the intervention of the state in social welfare.

The extent to which such consensus on the growth of the state was embraced by a wider constituency than that of government is one of the problems considered later in this book. We move now to consider the apparent breakdown of this consensus in the years following 1975.

The demise of welfare statism?

As is made clear below, ideas about and the practice of social policy have been the subject of significant, some say radical, change between the mid-1970s and the present. The election of Mrs Thatcher as leader of the Conservative party in 1975 marked the beginning of a shift in the emphasis of Conservative economic and social policy. Three Conservative administrations headed by her introduced new (or reintroduced old) ideas about the role of government and state, and their relationship with civil society. As we will also see, those governments not only introduced new ideas but also attempted to shift the direction of social policy and the welfare state. With the fall of Mrs Thatcher in 1990 came the elevation of her protégé, John Major. Major's premiership has, according to some, seen the maturity of some Thatcherite social policies and the development of some new ones. This process is documented and analysed below (Chapter 7).

In 1979 the first of three Thatcher governments was elected. Its election manifesto drew extensively on the work of economists, philosophers and social scientists of the radical right (Hayek, 1944; Friedman, 1962; Powell, 1969; Joseph, 1972, 1976) as well as retaining some elements of the earlier Heathite consensus. Gradually, those consensus trails appear to have been removed as a form of 'new Conservatism' developed as the loadstone of government economic and social policy. The policies of Thatcher's governments have been seen by some as 'Powellism in government' (Barnett, 1984), nursed and developed into maturity by Sir Keith Joseph acting in the role of ideological commissar. The principles on which Thatcher's Conservatism were based seem to be threefold:

1. A need to reduce drastically government expenditure as the public sector is seen as a burden on wealth-creating sectors of the economy.
2. A firm control of the money supply is needed in order to restrain inflation.
3. A reduction or confinement of the role of government simply to that needed for the maintenance of conditions in which free markets may function properly.

Put quite simply, it was the enunciation of these principles and their partial, if not complete, translation into government policies which led to promotion of the idea that the British state, after three decades of interventionism, had been 'rolled back' or withdrawn from interference in the affairs of civil society. As we will see, changes occurred in the relationship between state and civil society during this period. An apparent consensus, however limited or extensive, was *seemingly* shattered. Government aims in this period differed from those of governments in the earlier post-war period, as witnessed by the following proposition by Joseph and Sumption:

> the aim must be to challenge one of the central prejudices of modern British politics, the belief that it is the proper function of the state to influence the redistribution of wealth for its own sake. (1979, p. 232)

Our goal of explaining state intervention in the post-1945 period – apparent consensus on growing state intervention, followed by apparent rupture of that consensus – will, however, be most aided not by a study of statements of intent but by a consideration of empirical realities. It is therefore to those realities that we must now move.

Prelude: the early 1970s

As early as the beginning of the 1970s, the post-war settlement on economic and social intervention appeared vulnerable. Although the political rhetoric of government was still couched in terms of repairing rather than challenging that settlement, policy changes were occurring which appeared to be portents of a fundamental shift in the role and functions of the British state. The Heath Conservative government (1970–4) flirted with post-Keynesian economics and a reduction in state activity in the economy. So-called lame-duck industries were refused further government subsidy and allowed to go to the wall in the eponymous *Selsdon Man* period before a reversion to the consensus management of earlier periods reasserted itself in the latter stages of that government. The Wilson government (1974–6) appeared to abandon, once elected, the commitment to full employment on which the post-war settlement had been built (Riddell, 1983). It was in the years following 1975, however, that the interventionist state *appeared* to be 'undergoing an abrupt and fundamental reversal of its whole direction' (Taylor-Gooby, 1985, p. 12).

1975–9: the winds of change?

This short period of time is a particularly interesting one. For these four short years a Labour government presided over an economy sliding into reverse. Unemployment rates were rising alarmingly, if not as spectacularly as in the early 1980s: inflation at times seemed apparently uncontrollable (for a contemporary account of the period see Sked and Cook, 1979, ch. 12 and for interesting analyses of this period see Morgan, 1990 and Williamson, 1990). Economic crisis followed economic crisis and industrial conflict reached new heights culminating in the 'winter of discontent' of 1978–9. During the winter months of 1978–9 the trade union movement rejected government policies, particularly those on wage restraint, aimed at dealing with Britain's economic crisis and mounted a campaign of industrial action which played a part in the defeat of the then Labour government in the 1979 General Election. If there has been a fundamental shift in the nature and scope of state intervention in British society, then this period may be regarded by later commentators as a period of transition from a consensus on state involvement and growing state expenditure to one in which fundamental conflict characterised the debate on the role of the state in civil society and the degree of economic intervention and expenditure acceptable in a modern society. Riddell, commenting on this period argues 'if there has been a Thatcher experiment it was launched by Denis Healey' (1983, p. 59).

During this period government policies on state expenditure and on state involvement in industry and the public sector of the economy seem to have reflected, on the one hand a commitment to the interventionist state which had been the political commonsense of the post-1945 period. On the other hand, economic policies also appeared to include elements which portended a future reduction in state activities.

Throughout this brief period, the Labour government attempted to implement Keynesian or neo-Keynesian economic policies to hold down unemployment. It also sanctioned and encouraged increased intervention by the state into other areas of economic management. In particular, the development of a 'social contract' between government and trade unions amounted to state intervention to control pay and prices and was, arguably, the high-tide mark of the interpenetration of state and civil society in Britain. In effect, at least for a short period, government and state offered, and the trade union movement (or at least its leaders) accepted, the role of a quasi-state agency, monitoring and, where possible, controlling increases in pay. On the other hand, it was this Labour government which introduced an economic strategy part of which was governed by monetarist principles. This development is amply described and analysed in a number of excellent texts (especially McLennan, *et al.*, 1984) but appears to have consisted of the following features:

(a) attempts to control the money supply (first introduced in 1975);
(b) attempts to reduce public expenditure, or at least to halt its rise;

(c) application of cash limits to public spending and to curb the
    Public Sector Borrowing Requirement.

These monetarist policies undoubtedly led to a reduction in state
provision in welfare services as in other services and have been
seen as paving the way for private provision and privatisation even
if that were not the political intention.

Some have argued that the monetarism of the Labour government in the mid-to-late 1970s should be seen as a politically expe-
dient response to external pressures rather than as a principled
abandonment of Keynesian economic precepts. Prime among
these external pressures were the requirements of the International Monetary Fund (IMF) in granting Britain a loan during the
sterling crisis of 1976 (Riddell, 1983, p. 59). They point to the
'uncertain mix of policies' (Riddell, 1983, p. 60), to monetarist
policies juggled alongside incomes policies and measures to hold
down unemployment. They contrast such an eclectic mix with the
straightforward monetarism of the later Thatcher governments. Be
that as it may, the winds of change in attitudes to state intervention
had started to blow during the Labour government of the late
1970s.

Changes were also occurring, of course, as a result of Mrs
Thatcher's leadership of the Conservative Party. Under her
leadership, policy prescriptions here, as in social policy, tilted
markedly to the right. Whether they precipitated a sea change in
state activity in the 1980s is quite another question.

The rhetoric and reality of the new Conservatism

In May 1979 a Conservative government was elected in Britain
apparently pledged to political philosophies and practices quite
different from those of the governments of the post-war consensus
period. The new Prime Minister and her senior colleagues presented a programme of change for Britain which had been developed over some years and which owed much to the writers of
the radical right. The aim of the 'new Conservatism' was to shatter
what was seen as the post-war consensus on state interventionism,
mixed economy and welfare or, in the words of one Thatcherite, to
reject the 'false trails of Butskellism' (Lawson, 1981) and to create
a new consensus based on quite different principles. Deliberate

attempts were to be made to shift the frontiers between the public and private sectors of the British economy, to introduce policies which would stimulate private enterprise and to encourage the creation of a strong private sector in welfare. The proposed principles which would guide policy-making were regarded by the new government – and by many contemporary writers (Hall, 1979; Leonard, 1979; Gamble, 1979, 1980) – as the antithesis of previously dominant consensus principles. Specifically these new guiding principles included:

(a) a commitment to large scale state intervention in social and economic life being replaced by a commitment to a market economy (Howe, 1983);

(b) a commitment to the authority of the state being replaced by a commitment to the rule of law (Howe, 1983);

(c) a commitment to large scale state intervention in welfare being replaced by a commitment only to a *residual* welfare state (Boyson, 1971; Joseph, 1976; Seldon, 1977, 1981; Harris and Seldon, 1987).

Political orthodoxies about the relationship between the British state and civil society appeared to have been cast aside. The new Conservatives diagnosed state control and/or regulation of industry, industrial development and industrial relations as having sapped the initiative of private entrepreneurs and as having led to economic decline. Industry and economy needed to be freed of the fetters of state controls and subject only to the regulation of the market. The economic system, if it were to generate wealth and freedom, needed to be developed around the principle of voluntary exchange.

The growth of the state, and particularly the growth of welfare bureaucracies, protective legislation and the like, had elevated the authority of the state over people's lives to unacceptable proportions (Powell, 1969). The new Conservative proposals included ones concerned with severely limiting the state's paternalistic role and reinstating the rule of law as the primary institution regulating social and economic life (Howe, 1983).

The erstwhile political orthodoxy – of large scale state provision and control of welfare – was also to be challenged. The 'nanny-state' was to be rolled back. Responsibility for the provision of welfare was to be put back in its rightful place – with the individual, the family and the community – and large areas of welfare provision were to be privatised (Conservative Party, 1979).

In short, the new Conservatives at the beginning of the 1980s promised a transformation of the relationships between state and society – a transformation that was to be based on the economic principle of sound money and the moral principles of individual freedom and individual responsibility. In their analysis, consensus, state interventionist Britain had created a coercive state in an attempt to redistribute income, wealth and life chances. That coercive state had, at one and the same time destroyed freedom and the economic growth which was the precondition of redistribution. The new order – based on a sense of personal responsibility, a concept of community self-help and on a concept of individual rather than collective justice (B. Griffiths, 1983, p. 7) – presumed, in contrast,

> a certain kind and degree of inequality. . . . If society wants to preserve economic freedom it cannot predetermine equality which can only be achieved by coercion and therefore against freedom.
> (B. Griffiths, 1983, p. 9)

So, if this was the rhetoric of change, what have been the empirical realities of state intervention in Britain since 1979? This is a question to which we turn in the next chapter.

CHAPTER 2

Social policy in the 1980s and 1990s

1979-93: the new Conservative experiment

The 1979 General Election marks the start of what some (Riddell, 1983; Hall and Jacques, 1985) have seen as the 'Thatcher Experiment'. The task before us is to describe and begin to analyse the significance of that experiment.

The first administration

The 1979 Conservative government came to power at a time when unemployment was rising, industrial relations were sour, public expenditure had been cut and the British economy was in freefall. Its reaction was to attempt to redefine the appropriate role of government in a modern society. Social policy was one of the central targets of that redefinition.

The end of full employment

Although unemployment had risen alarmingly under the Wilson–Callaghan governments (1974–79), the first Thatcher government appears to have accepted it as a policy in its own right. As has already been observed, the outgoing Labour government had, in 1976, accepted the conditions laid down by the IMF in return for substantial loans. These conditions had included the explicit abandonment of Keynesian budget management and this had, along with pursuant cuts in public expenditure, created higher unemployment.

Mrs Thatcher's first government adopted policies which seemed to signal an end to the formal commitment to full employment. As early as 1979, the Chancellor reduced rates of income tax, but, unlike President Reagan in the United States, the government was unwilling to rely on the Laffer Doctrine and wait for improvements in government revenue that might arise from increased individual incomes. Instead, the UK government financed its cuts in direct taxation by increasing indirect taxation (including a near doubling of value added tax and an increase in social security tax). The result of this strategy was to make spending more difficult, rather than easier, a condition which generated higher unemployment. That this was a conscious strategy is in little doubt. The Prime Minister, herself already a monetarist of the Friedman school, had earlier signalled her agreement with the economist's view that unemployment was a necessary component of a low inflation policy (Sullivan, 1989; Glennerster and Midgley, 1991). What is less clear is whether the government recognised at this point that the situation would be further exacerbated by other economic and social policies that they were to adopt as part of the same struggle to keep inflation low. These policies included having a high interest rate and further reduction in public expenditure (especially on capital projects). The result of this combination of policies was to push Britain into recession and to increase unemployment further.

This form of *machismo monetarism*, 'if it isn't hurting then it isn't working' (Thatcher speech, n.d.), had two obvious effects. First, it elevated unemployment to the status of policy instrument. Second, it led to the accumulation of a budget surplus. These policy developments in the first Thatcher term mark the unambiguous ascendancy of radical right thinking in government. Though this was particularly the case in relation to economic policy, it had, of course, clear social policy implications. Cuts in public expenditure ate into the fabric of the welfare state, while consistently high unemployment rates would make the financing of welfare more difficult. The threefold increase in social security payments between 1979 and 1982, a direct result of the increase in unemployment, served to reinforce this view.

The first major change associated with Thatcher governments was thus an abandonment of the principle of full employment. Implicit in this abandonment was a rejection of the Beveridge principles that was to be made explicit later. Beveridge had correctly assumed that the successful administration of a social security system and the maintenance of a welfare state were dependent on full employment (Beveridge, 1942; Hill, 1990; Sullivan, 1992). Without full employment, paying for welfare became an onerous burden on government and people. The use of unemployment as a policy instrument would therefore create a fiscal crisis which was, as we shall see later, followed and supplemented by questions about the welfare state's legitimacy.

A further intention of the conscious use of unemployment by government was, at least according to some (see, Walker, 1983; Sullivan, 1989 for example), the suppression of the low pay lobby. The argument here is that the threat of unemployment would tend to extinguish efforts to improve the conditions of those workers on low pay, therefore satisfying the wish for a 'high technology, low pay economy' (Lawson, 1981).

Thus beginnings of a new Conservative social policy were emerging during Thatcher's first term of government. The clearest feature of this embryonic social policy was the acceptance or use of high unemployment.

Public expenditure fettered

The second major ambition of the government during this first term was, as we have noted above, the constraint of public expenditure. As a strategy, restriction on public expenditure was seen as both fiscally necessary and socially desirable. Its fiscal attraction was the obvious one of arresting and reversing the upward trend in expenditure on the welfare state. Its social desirability lay in the fact that less expenditure on welfare meant, or would ultimately mean, less welfare. Given the Thatcher government's views, borrowed from Hayek, Powell and Joseph (see Sullivan, 1989), that the welfare state had created a dependency culture and a work-shy population, public expenditure cuts offered one of the routes to a revitalised, individualistic society with only residual state welfare functions.

In the event the strategy met with only limited success. Local government spending on education, housing and personal social services was severely curbed but the savings made on welfare state spending were more than accounted for by the 300 per cent increase in social security expenditure between 1980 and 1982. That expenditure was necessitated, of course, because of the pursuit of monetarist macroeconomic objectives. Attempts were made, at least in the social security system, to square the circle. These attempts included:

(a) the abolition of some social security benefits;
(b) changes in the basis for entitlement to others; and
(c) reduction in the real value of selected benefits.

The abolition of the Earnings Related Unemployment Supplement, which introduced the principle of graduated unemployment benefits, is an example of attempts to make savings by the removal of a benefit. This benefit, introduced in 1966 by a Labour government, was intended to cushion those made temporarily unemployed during a period of rapid industrial change. It was abolished in 1982.

The strategy of reducing the value of some social security benefits was adopted in the decision in 1980 to de-index long-term benefits. In 1974, the then Labour government had linked annual increases in long-term benefits – such as pensions – to whichever was the higher of measures of price inflation or earnings. This was replaced by a decision to relate the benefit to price inflation only and was fully enacted in 1983 (see below) along with further changes in the way that price inflation was calculated. This ensured that further disadvantages accrued to claimants and further savings were made by government (Sullivan, 1989, p. 44). These savings amounted, in the first year of operation, to a sum in the region of £500 million (Riddell, 1983; Sullivan, 1989).

Some have also argued that the policy choice of de-indexing *long-term* benefits had ideological as well as fiscal appeal (Sullivan, 1989; 1992; Mishra, 1990). This attraction, if it existed, lay in the fortuitous division of benefit recipients into the potentially productive groups, whose benefits were not de-indexed, on the one hand and the unproductive, including the elderly, on the other.

Another strategy also possessing dual fiscal and ideological appeals was that of effecting reduction in the level of benefit without making overt cuts. One of the most obvious examples of this strategy was the decision in 1982, to tax unemployment benefit. The strategy here was, at one and the same time, to recoup revenue for the Exchequer and to ensure that the level of unemployment benefit was pegged below the wages of low-paid workers. Thus, not only would fiscal imperatives be satisfied. A distinction between the working poor and the non-working poor would be constructed and the operation of a principle of 'less eligibility' reintroduced (Johnson, 1990; Sullivan, 1992).

However, in the early years the Thatcher government only succeeded in devoting a higher proportion of gross domestic product (GDP) to welfare spending. This was, as has already been noted, almost entirely the result of trebling unemployment benefit costs during this period. Indeed, the effect of high unemployment throughout the first two Thatcher Administrations was to have the effect (further cuts in public spending notwithstanding) of modifying the goals of government from reducing the proportion of GDP expended on welfare to arresting the upward trend. This might be regarded as a classic example of an unexpected disjuncture between early policy intentions and early and later outcomes (Johnson, 1990; Glennerster and Midgley, 1991; Hills, 1991).

National Health Service or health care insurance?

Between 1979 and 1982, the Administration considered alternative forms of health cover to the National Health Service. It is well known that Mrs Thatcher and her senior ministers and advisers considered the option of replacing the NHS, with its guarantee of treatment free at the point of use, with a system of health insurance (Sullivan, 1989, 1992). In the event, this option was abandoned in 1982 after a fact-finding mission to the United States by the then Secretary of State for Health, Patrick Jenkin. Structural changes in the NHS were to be delayed for a further eight years.

What seems clear is that a new Conservative social policy was beginning to emerge during the first Thatcher administration. That embryonic social policy suggested the replacement of a collectivist consensus by an emphasis on small government and individual responsibility. That its fiscal effects differed, to some degree, from policy intention was in part due to increased unemployment and the failure of this early government to alter substantially the principles governing the receipt of benefit. Radical changes would await the election of the second and third administrations.

1983–90: a radical approach to social policy?

During the two administrations which followed 1983, the tentative steps to retrench social policy that had occurred in the first term gave way to a more sure-footed attempt to tackle what was seen as an overweening welfare state. In fact, structural changes in welfare were attempted.

Attempts at radical change

The first social policy area targeted for change was the social security system. From the government's vantage point there were good reasons for this. In the first place, spending on social security amounted to approximately half of all social spending; in 1983, it was the fastest growing element of the UK welfare state (Minford, 1983; Hill, 1990; Hills, 1990; Glennerster and Midgley, 1991), particularly as a result of still increasing unemployment. This circumstance was exacerbated by relatively generous levels of pensions for a growing elderly population that had been introduced by the last Labour government. Government therefore decided to act firmly in an attempt to slash spending on social security and thus move some way towards its welfare state spending targets.

There might have been another reason for seeking to overhaul the social security system. This was the problem of the 'poverty trap'. Radical right economists who had the ear of government (see Minford, 1983, for instance) were concerned about the alleged propensity of the system to act as a work disincentive.

The argument went something like this. Previous Labour and Conservative governments had pitched benefit levels too close to the wage levels of lower paid workers. Consequently, benefit claimants had little or no incentive to find low-paid work. Indeed, Minford comes close to presenting this alleged system-induced work-shy behaviour as the major contributory factor in rising unemployment (1983). This situation was compounded by the fact that receipt of mandatory benefit acted as a 'passport' to certain discretionary benefits that either disappeared or were taxed pound for pound once the beneficiary found work, and to free services in other areas of welfare (optical, dental and school meals services, for example). Government, its neo-liberal supporters and, indeed, the political left found the existence of a poverty trap an undesirable state of affairs, though right and left differed on the nature of policy solutions to the problem (Minford, 1983; Walker and Walker, 1987).

The solution adopted by the government to the problem of social security had two parts, one procedural and the other structural. Its first action was to alter the basis on which all benefits would be calculated. Since the 1950s, even those benefits which were not index-linked had been uprated annually in line with rises in the general standard of living. In 1983 this changed and was replaced by a previously agreed principle of uprating in line with annual increases in prices only. The outcome of this move was to increase the relative income gap between claimants and those in work. As wages in the real economy increased the relative value of benefits fell. The group hit hardest were the unemployed. Indeed this was part of the policy strategy. Unemployment benefit fell in value when compared with wages. Not only this, but as stated above, it became tax-liable. As a result of these changes, benefits were worth only one-eighth of average earnings by the end of the decade.

The second part of government strategy was intended to be considerably more significant, though it simply extended the logic of earlier decisions on benefit levels. In 1984, the then Secretary of State for Health and Social Security announced the government's intention to mount a detailed review of the social security system. Though the review took two years and was intended to replace the Beveridge principles with something closer to the views of radical right economists, its outcome was somewhat more modest. In the first place, the intentions of government had included the phased replacement of the State Earnings Related Pension Scheme (SERPS) by private provision. In the end, the reviewers concluded that this was impossible. The privatisation proposal assumed that instead of contributing to a state scheme, individuals would make compulsory contributions to a private scheme and would thus ultimately rid government of responsibility for older people. This policy proposal was opposed not only by the poverty lobby, to which the government had stopped listening anyway, but also by the private insurance industry. The insurance business took the view that coverage of the whole of pensioners' insurance needs was a risky proposition and preferred to remain as providers of top-up pension schemes to state pensioners (Hill, 1990; Johnson, 1990). Facing up to this, changes in this aspect of social security have merely meant that the state scheme has been made less fiscally attractive and that tax incentives have been introduced to encourage the taking up of private pension schemes.

Other outcomes of the review included the replacement of Supplementary Benefit by Income Support, of Family Income Support by Family Credit and of one-off discretionary payments by a Social Fund dealing largely in loan-making. The effect of these changes has been a meaner and leaner social security system. They do not, however, amount to the replacement of Beveridge that the government appeared to promise and that many feared.

The relative failure of the social security reviews in changing the underlying principles led one radical right commentator to argue that radical change is best managed in two phases. The first phase involves changes in the administration of public services to bring them closer to the ethos of the private corporation. The second phase, that of privatisation of public services, is thus made easier (Seldon, 1986). This appears to be a strategy that Thatcher governments adopted, purposely or accidentally in some other social policy areas (see below).

Radical change effected?

More significant success was managed by government in other areas of social policy. This was particularly the case in the third Thatcher term. Though even here there were instances of spectacular failure.

The Conservative manifesto for the 1987 General Election (Conservative Party, 1987) seemed to suggest that the party was willing to go for broke in introducing radical social policy changes. Here we will consider four policy innovations, three of which were prefigured in the manifesto. They are the introduction of the Community Charge, the Housing Act (1988), the creation of grant maintained status ('opting-out') for state schools and the National Health Service reforms.

The Community Charge, or the poll tax as it is better known, was introduced by government as a replacement for local rates. It required all but a small minority of adults to make a flat rate contribution to local authorities and thus differed from the previous rating system in that it took the individual rather than the household as the unit for taxpaying purposes. One of the effects of this was that the tax liability of many households was increased and, given that the scheme was flat-rate, failed to take into account the taxpayer's ability to pay. The introduction of the poll tax was seen by government as serving several functions:

(a) the abolition of a rating system universally regarded as inequitable;
(b) the introduction of a notion of fairness in the payment of local tax (a household with one member had previously payed the same rates as a household with many members); and
(c) the notion of local accountability (it was expected that poll taxpayers would punish any council which overspent and therefore made its local taxpayers liable for a greater poll tax burden).

In fact the experiment turned out to be an almost total political disaster. The tax was unpopular. Citizens faced with high tax bills in the first year of its operation blamed not allegedly spendthrift local authorities but the government which introduced the tax. Neither was this hostility diminished by the decision of government to increase its grants to local councils in the second year of the poll tax and thus make poll tax bills smaller. As a result, following the resignation of Prime Minister Thatcher in 1990, the government gave notice of its intention to ditch the system and replace it with a council tax.

Further failure, or at least relative failure, attended the implementation of the Housing Act 1988 and the Education Reform Act of the same year. Or so it seemed at the time.

The Housing Act permitted council housing to be transferred from the control of local councils to private sector management bodies if the tenants of a street, block or estate so wished. Though government loaded the policy dice in favour of such opt-out schemes – a failure to vote in a tenants' ballot on transfer of control was originally counted as an assenting voice – few landlords and relatively few housing associations indicated their wish to take over erstwhile council housing.

Initially, at least, the picture was the same in education. One of the key elements of the Education Reform Act (1988) empowered parents to vote to transfer the status of local education authority (LEA) schools to that of grant maintained schools funded directly by the Secretary of State for Education (for more detailed descriptions of the process of transfer, see Simon, 1988; Sullivan, 1989). In the first two years of this scheme only sixty UK schools opted to transfer status, and in some places moves to grant maintenance were resisted equally strongly by Conservative councillors as by Labour councillors (Glennerster and Midgley, 1991; Sullivan, 1991).

However, there was a clear and resounding policy success during this third term. It was one which was not even hinted at in the Conservative manifesto for the 1987 General Election. This is all the more startling because the changes wrought were little short of revolutionary. I am referring, of course, to the results of the NHS review in the late 1980s. The popular affection for the NHS remained unvanquished during the Thatcher years. It seemed to be as much part of the furniture of British life as fish and chips and the monarchy. Certainly, this popularity remained undimmed at the end of the decade (Jowell *et al.*, 1989). None the less, political circumstances of the government's own making conspired to push reform of the NHS to the top of the policy agenda.

The NHS had been subject to cash constraints for much of the Thatcher period. These constraints contributed, in 1988, to an embarrassing series of exposés of seriously ill children being turned away from intensive therapy units because of staff shortages. Mrs Thatcher's characteristic political luck deserted her over this issue and she was harried successfully over a number of weeks by the Labour Opposition, who reminded her that she had once promised that 'the National Health Service is safe with us'. Though her predicament was uncharacteristic, her eventual policy response bore the hallmarks of a premier used to making policy on the hoof. She announced the establishment of a comprehensive review of the NHS and proudly declared that all policy options, including the abolition of the NHS, would be on the table. If the NHS was not working then maybe it needed to be replaced by a different system of health care.

The review, which was charged to report to the Prime Minister within the year, received submissions from all political directions. Some advice from the political right focused on ways of running down the NHS gradually and replacing it with a system of private health insurance (see Pirie and Butler, 1988). Another suggestion was that the NHS should be replaced by health maintenance organisations (HMOs) on the American model (Goldsmith and Willetts, 1988). The radical right seemed intent on taking Reagan's

America as the pattern for a future British health system but most
of the other evidence submitted to the reviewers was supportive of
the NHS. This evidence drew attention to underfunding of the
service and suggested that this state of affairs lay at the heart of the
problem. Some commentators suggested judicious experimentation within the existing structures of the welfare state (Barr *et al.*,
1988) but few outside the right-wing think tanks suggested that the
NHS was a suitable case for surgery.

The strategy of abolition and replacement was dropped by the
review team almost immediately. There appear to be two reasons
for this. The first was timescale. The reviewers had been instructed
by the Prime Minister to report in no more than one year and this
all but precluded in their minds – if not in hers – a thorough review
of the evidence on the viability of alternative systems to the NHS.
The second reason, and one familiar to students of social policy-
making was the Treasury. Quite simply, the Department was convinced that to follow the American pattern of third party private
health insurance would be to court the disaster that had befallen
the American health care system, namely the explosion of health
care costs which had been witnessed by Jenkin earlier in the decade (Barr *et al.*, 1988; Leathard, 1991). The structural changes
suggested by the right wing were therefore rejected with the aid of
the conservative impulses of the Treasury mandarins. Be that as it
may radical structural changes were proposed by the reviewers
and, after refinement, implemented.

The review recommended the introduction of an internal or
quasi-market in the NHS. The basic right of the patient to treatment free at the point of use was to remain as was the method of
funding the service through taxation. However, the reviewers suggested a fundamental internal reorganisation. The idea was that
district health authorities (DHAs) should commission services
from whichever hospital was regarded as providing the best quality
services. In other words, hospitals were to compete with each other
for business. A market was to be created in the NHS in which
efficient, good quality hospitals would be rewarded with DHA
contracts. The bracing winds of competition would also act as a
spur to less efficient under-performing hospitals in that the loss of
contracts would impel them to improve performance in order to
win contracts in the future. These recommendations were, of
course, music to the Prime Minister's ears. They were consistent

with the new Conservatism of which she was the prominent public promoter and were consonant with the radical right belief that competition improved efficiency and performance. The idea itself was not new and had been floated by a leading American advocate of managed competition on a visit to the United Kingdom in 1985 (Enthoven, 1985).

The concept of 'managed competition' was at the heart of the White Paper, *Working for Patients* (Department of Health, 1989) and of the National Health and Community Care Act which was given the royal assent in 1990. DHAs, instead of providing, managing and funding all services in a given geographical area became, simply, the purchasers of those services. What emerged from 1 April 1991 was a system which bore close resemblance to the 'preferred provider model' adopted in the American Medicare system and in private health insurance schemes in the United States.

DHAs were expected to purchase services not only from NHS hospitals in their own area but from NHS hospitals, emerging NHS trusts (see Sullivan, 1992) and private hospitals. The NHS, which had always had elements of a mixed economy of welfare about it (Sullivan, 1987), moved towards a market model – even if that model was to be managed rather than entirely free.

Further Americanisation was proposed in relation to the organisation of general practitioner (GP) services. The reforms introduced the possibility, opposed by the general public and initially by the BMA and the doctors, for GPs to be part of fund-holding practices. As a result of this change, doctors in larger practices could opt to receive a budget from the Department of Health to purchase services for their patients (Leathard, 1991; Glennerster and Midgley, 1991; Sullivan, 1992). In this they were to behave similarly to HMOs in the United States.

The introduction of the internal market constitutes a major change in policy direction. In implementation, however, this revolutionary policy change may have proved less startling than might have been expected by government.

The problem about inserting quasi-American structures into the NHS was, of course, the differences between health markers in the United Kingdom and the United States. The excess supply of beds in American hospitals makes genuine competition possible. In the United Kingdom, by contrast, there is a shortage of supply-side provision, most of which is – in any case – concentrated in district general hospitals. Consequently, following the enactment of the National Health and Community Care Act, patterns of contract between DHAs and local hospitals remained largely unchanged. DHAs behaved as they had always done when commissioning services but did so in a way more closely defined by the Department of Health.

The intervention of fund-holding GP practices in the market had a potentially more profound effect. Giving local doctors the power and the resources to purchase care theoretically brings service accountability closer to the patient. It also gives local doctors the potential to be more careful about their choice of patients, the fear being that iller and more expensive patients might come to be seen as unwelcome burdens on the practice budget.

We might conclude that the NHS reforms failed fully to introduce a radical right approach to welfarism. Markets were introduced but, in the short term at least, refused to behave like markets. To come to this judgement only would, however, be to miss a fundamental point not lost on radical right lobbyists outside government. The point is this: the introduction of the internal market moved the NHS closer to a private model. The further introduction of NHS Trusts and of GP fund-holding has reinforced this trend and, taken together, the reforms made it easier to privatise the service in the future. Is this the two-stage process to which Seldon (1986) refers? (For further discussion on this, see Chapter 4.)

In late 1990 Mrs Thatcher was toppled as leader of the Conservative Party and as Prime Minister following a 'palace coup'. During her tenure as premier, her governments had attempted radical and structural changes to the welfare state. While succeeding in reversing the upward trend in welfare spending – expenditure on health, education and social benefits had decreased from a high of 11.2 per cent of GDP in 1985 to 6.9 per cent in 1990 (National Institute for Economic and Social Research, 1991, p. 115) – and in getting the NHS reforms on to the statute book, those governments were certainly less than immediately successful in rolling the state back from welfare. While it is beyond doubt that those governments intended to smash the previous welfarist consensus, the indications are that it was less than completely successful in that intention. That, at least, is one interpretation. Another, while acknowledging that these years represent an incomplete revolution in social policy, sees the changes introduced by the Thatcher governments as pragmatic first and second steps towards the radical right utopia of stateless welfare. We move, in the next section, to consider the evidence for both these hypotheses provided by the years 1990–1993.

1990–93: development of the Thatcher project or its demise?

In November 1990, following political turmoil in the Conservative Party, Margaret Thatcher resigned as Prime Minister and was replaced by John Major. Though the new Prime Minister had been Thatcher's Chancellor of the Exchequer, political pundits opined on whether his accession would mean a break with the policy principles with which she (and, incidentally, he) had been associated or whether continuity would characterise the policy agenda in social policy and elsewhere. This was not, of course, merely journalistic puff. Early in his first term as Prime Minister, Major, declared his political aspirations to include the creation of a classless society. He did not mean the same by this, of course, as had Karl Marx! Rather, he was talking about the creation of a society in which personal effort and equality of opportunity became political bedfellows in the project of making Britain a society 'at peace with itself'. Surely, then, the policy agenda and policy intentions were to change. Would not the creation of a harmonious Britain depend, in part, on government following a different social policy trajectory? Perhaps the Major premiership would mark a break with the policies and policy aspirations of Conservative governments since 1979.

Words are, of course, sometimes deceptive and the words of career politicians are often open to a multiplicity of interpretations. There is, on one reading at least, evidence to suggest that a social policy audit of the two Major administrations implies continuity and development of Thatcherite policies rather than a disjuncture with them.

Health policy and the Major governments
The Major governments have introduced no significant new policies in the health field. Neither, however, do they seem to have

deviated from the course charted for them by the now Lady Thatcher. Indeed, secretaries of state in these administrations have energetically implemented policies emerging at the butt end of the Thatcher years. The idea and practice of an internal market has remained at the heart of policy on the NHS and the movement of NHS hospitals to Trust status has accelerated and been robustly encouraged by both of Major's Secretaries of State for Health. In the run up to the 1992 General Election, William Waldegrave, Major's then urbane Health Minister, indicated that there was little alternative for district hospitals and other health units but to become NHS Trusts. If the Conservatives were elected, he suavely reassured, there would be no attempt to compel units to opt out of DHA control. Rather, NHS Trusts would simply be the government's 'preferred policy option, our preferred model' (*The Guardian*, 6 March 1992). The political message was clear, however, and health service managers needed no help in decoding it. For Waldegrave had made clear a point reinforced by his successor, Virginia Bottomley. Trusts would, at least in the short run, be the beneficiaries of greater resources than non-Trust hospitals. The effect, of course, has been to translate the trickle of hospitals applying for Trust status before the election into a flood. The same is the case with the GP fund-holding scheme, the entry criteria of which have been made easier by government.

It might, therefore, be reasonable to conclude that, in health at least, Conservative governments in the early 1990s have remained faithful to the policy principles of the Thatcher years. More than this, they seem to have experienced no discomfort in propelling those policy principles into life. By 1993, in excess of half of the United Kingdom's hospitals have become Trusts or have declared an interest in doing so within the year (Department of Health, 1993). A similar picture is emerging in relation to GP fund-holding. Structural changes to the NHS, started by the Thatcher governments, seem to have been developed and intensified under Major – but how radical are these changes politically and ideologically?

Measured against the original thoughts of the first Thatcher government or the advice of early radical right privatisers (Harris and Seldon, 1979), the changes are much less than right-wing Conservatives hoped for and many non-Conservatives feared. A National Health Service funded out of taxation remains in place. Despite the growth of private health care provision (Higgins, 1988, 1990; Johnson, 1990; Leathard, 1991; Sullivan, 1992), encouraged by government and further fostered by the assumption that DHAs will now buy some services from the private sector, NHS hospitals, Trusts or otherwise, remain the preponderant providers of health care.

Privatisation of the Service has not occurred. Perhaps Conservative governments in the 1990s, like their counterparts in the 1980s, have judged such a dramatic change in policy politically dangerous. Certainly, as we shall see later, abolition of the NHS would prove less than popular with the electorate. None the less, the change in policy direction has been significant. First, the service monopoly previously held by the NHS has been broken: private health care still remains a small part of total health care provision but the principle of a mixed economy of provision has been conceded. Second, the introduction of a quasi-market in health has moved the NHS nearer to the private model and has made privatisation of the service in future a much shorter step.

Education policy in the early 1990s
There is an essentially similar story to tell in relation to education policy. Policy changes in education came thick and fast in the Thatcher years: parental preference, the reintroduction of formal testing, the introduction of a national curriculum, the encouragement of efficiency measures, and greater competition in higher education and so on (Sullivan, 1989; Johnson, 1991; Jones, 1991). The Major governments have introduced no new policy trajectories but have implemented these earlier policy changes with vigour. The grant maintained status option opened to schools as a result of the Education Reform Act (1988) yielded less than impressive results up to 1992. Indeed, in its first two years of operation the response from schools was derisory. However, during the General Election campaign in 1992, the then Secretary of State for Education made it clear (in terms which strikingly resembled Waldegrave's words about NHS Trusts) that, if returned, the government would prefer schools to become grant maintained rather than continuing in LEA control. Following that election, the dam has burst and large numbers of schools have declared their wish to transfer status. It is estimated that by 1996 over 80 per cent of schools will have severed their links with LEAs (Aitken, 1992).

The Thatcher governments' concern with competition in the higher education sector has been acknowledged and acted upon. This is seen most sharply in the implementation by the second Major administration of an earlier policy proposal to dissolve the binary line in this sector. Accordingly, since 1992, erstwhile poly-technics which meet certain eligibility criteria have been allowed to transfer to the university sector. One of the reasons behind this move was that the new universities had developed as successful polytechnics by adopting market values. As a result they had often been more effective than established universities in attracting non-government funds for applied research and consultancy. The inser-tion of these institutions into an enlarged university sector would, it was hoped, encourage the old universities to compete for con-tracts in the real world of the market.

There were, of course, other equally important policy intentions behind this particular initiative. Two which are of prime import-ance were a concern with educational opportunity and an interest in efficiency. The nature of both these concerns owed much to the political philosophy which had nurtured Thatcherism and appears to have been a significant influence on the Major governments.

First is educational opportunity. In words reminiscent of the intellectual architect of post-war social democracy (see Crosland, 1974), the Major government, like the Thatcher governments be-fore it, has declared an interest in increasing access to higher edu-cation. The political motives behind increased access have, however, been quite different from those embraced by social democrats. While the impetus from social democracy for emphasis on equality of educational opportunity was due to a belief that modification of the inequalities in educational opportunity would have a carry-through effect into the managed labour market, con-temporary Conservatism appears to dance to a different political drum. Here, the attraction of increasing access to higher education appears to be a belief that government should act through educa-tion to increase the number of people equipped to compete in an unmanaged market economy. That is to say that, whereas the prin-ciple of equality of educational opportunity had previously been associated by social democracy with sister concerns for a labour market policy (Furniss and Tilton, 1979; Sullivan, 1992), the Con-servative emphasis on increased access appears to be connected with a desire to increase the numbers of citizens equipped to face the rigours of unmanaged capitalism. In any case, there are concerns that increasing access to higher education, whether through the enlargement of the university sector or by other means, is likely to be unsuccessful in expanding the pool of students benefiting from high quality education. Rather, say some, the outcome is likely to be the lowering of academic standards as higher education institutions seek to reach their targets for increased recruitment set by government. Arguably, then, the outcome of this policy emphasis, whatever its intention, is to decrease access to quality education.

The concern with efficiency which has been associated with dissolving the binary line can be expressed simply. The erstwhile polytechnics, though administered for most of their existence by LEAs, were seen as having secured their continuation in part by the adoption of efficiency strategies familiar in the world beyond the ivory tower (performance-related pay, performance reviews and the like). One of the outcomes hoped for from a merger of the new and old universities, was the permeation into the system as a whole of the attitudes behind these strategies.

The changes in education occurring in the period now considered, appear to some to have been momentous. Indeed, they may turn out so to be. It may be that grant maintained status in the school sector is a Trojan Horse bearing the threat of later complete privatisation. Changes in the higher education sector may well transform the nature of degree and post-degree education. It is still too soon to say. What can be said is that, inasmuch as government education policy represents a radical break with post-war consensus politics, the impetus for change came from a policy environment created by its predecessors. Conservative governments since 1990 have merely – though importantly – acted to encourage the widespread adoption of policy strategies in education set in place before the downfall of the previous Prime Minister.

In health and education, then, there looks to be no sign of demise of the Thatcherite social policy project. Indeed, in areas such as 'school opt-outs' and the creation of NHS Trusts, the Major administrations appear to have breathed life into Thatcher policy reforms. As we have already seen, the Thatcher governments of the 1980s had mixed fortunes in implementing post-consensus social policies. As we shall see below, in some policy areas at least, this led to rethinking the policy agenda. However, in the two areas

reviewed above, political principles establis
regimes have been fostered and nurtured.

Rethinking the policy agenda
There is some evidence that the Major gov
thought aspects of the Thatcher social policy ag
Shortly after the replacement of Mrs Thatch   ... ivlinis-
ter, the new Major cabinet made plans to replace the Community
Charge (poll tax) with a council tax which, it is believed, takes
more account of a citizen's ability to pay and partly reverts to the
principle of taxing according to property value. This new scheme,
implemented from 1993, and the policy process which created it
were in no small measure a response to public outcry that sometimes bordered on civil disobedience against the poll tax. Sufficient
taxpayers refused to pay as to create a crisis in local authority
finances, and general displeasure with the policy led government
to conclude that there was no political alternative but to remove it.
There are also indications that new thinking is taking place in
relation to the social security system. Once more, this review of
previous policy seems to have been forced on government. The
Fowler Review, as we have already seen, was nowhere near as
radical in its outcome as had been intended. Moreover, since the
implementation of the Fowler system, additional problems have
become apparent:

1. Administrative costs have remained high (and higher than in
   any other area of state welfare).
2. There have been runaway costs in certain benefit areas, particularly invalidity benefit which GPs appear to be sanctioning
   as an alternative to unemployment benefit, which is paid at a
   lower rate.
3. The Social Fund, by which local offices administer loans for
   one-off expenditure to claimants is budget limited and appears
   to work on a first-come first-served basis rather than on any
   objective need measuring footing and so on.

The result of these problems has been to raise the question of the
need for a 'new Beveridge' at the highest reaches of government.
Time will tell whether any changes in the social security system
amount to more than tinkering. From October 1993, right-wingers
within the Cabinet were mounting a robust attack on social

rity spending. Both the social security minister and the Secret-ry of State for Wales appeared to be suggesting savage cuts to, or the removal of, social security benefits to single parents.

The Major administrations and social policy

In summary, we might make the following observations about social policy developments since 1990. First, there has been a large degree of continuity between the welfare ideology and social policy innovations of the Thatcher and Major governments. Indeed, where policy revision has occurred, or is occurring, it appears to be a result of public political pressure or of fiscal and administrative crisis. Second, where there have been changes, there appears to be no consistency in policy direction. That is to say, although replacement of the Community Charge may come to be seen as a liberalisation of Thatcher policy, any future changes to the social security system may well have the effect of making it less generous than during the Thatcher years.

Social policy and new Conservatism: an appraisal

What then are we to make of the changes in social policy since the breakdown of post-war consensus? On one reading, the changes are less fundamental than new Conservatism promised: the structure of the welfare state remains largely, if not completely, intact; privatisation, though it has occurred, has been less extensive in outcome than in policy intention; the provision of welfare still appears to be a citizen's right. Read another way, the changes have been gradual but profound.

Long-term strategy and incremental change

A not implausible reading of the contemporary politics of social policy is to see continuity rather than conflict between the rhetoric of policy change and reality. Although the most radical policy intentions of recent Conservative governments have not been translated into policy outcomes at the first attempt, it is possible to discern the process as one where long-term strategy is the guiding principle behind incremental change.

Viewed from the 1990s, this might seem to be the ca:
principal welfare state areas. In housing and personal sc
vices, as in health education and social security, the accumulated
changes in policy direction have been significant.

Though the early rhetoric of rolling the state back from welfare
has not been fully realised, the welfare state of the 1990s more
fully resembles market organisations than would have seemed possible twenty years earlier. That recent Conservative administrations have, in large part, been the midwives of this change is not in
question. It is as true when we look at the governments headed by
Mr Major as when we consider the earlier Conservative administrations. Each of the five Conservative governments between
1979 and the early 1990s has engaged in incremental changes to the
fabric of welfare. By 1993, these increments have come to look
more and more like pieces in a strategic jigsaw puzzle. The ideas
behind this puzzle are considered more fully in later chapters.
Before we get there, however, we need to analyse the ideas behind
post-war welfare statism. It is to this task that we turn in the
following two chapters.

Understanding the state and social policy

CHAPTER 3

Understanding the modern British state

The primary concern of the opening chapters has been to map out the terrain of state involvement in British society during the past forty-five years or so. This chapter aims to construct a set of route maps to help us explore that post-war terrain. In Chapter 4 this undertaking is developed with specific reference to state intervention in social policy.

Three models of the British state and its involvement in social and economic life are reviewed here. This examination is both historical and topical. It considers erstwhile dominant or influential understandings of the state and then looks at how and why these approaches have been challenged in the last decade or so.

The erstwhile orthodoxy: social democracy and the state

For many post-war years, dominant models of the state and of its activities in civil society drew on the political theory of social democracy. This political strand, represented most clearly by the British Labour Party, generated a set of closely related perceptions about the nature and authority of state action.

Close attention is paid here to the work of a number of writers, many associated with the Labour Party in the 1950s and 1960s, who came to be seen as new revisionist thinkers.

The work of this group of Labour intellectuals, though clearly within the same political tradition, is diverse in its aims and intentions. Some of it consciously aims to provide a theory for social democracy in the late twentieth century (Crosland, 1956, 1974).

Some of it was intended to inform intra-party struggles within the Labour Party between its left and right wings (Crossman, 1950, 1952; Crosland, 1952, 1956, 1974; see also, Sullivan, 1992, 1994). Other work is more concerned with refining or updating the original revisionist theses developed during the 1950s (e.g. Williams, 1981). Taken together, this corpus of literature allows us to construct a social democratic perspective on the state and state intervention.

A transformed state

Much of the literature on the modern British state acknowledges that the post-war settlement, involving macro-level management of a mixed economy, and the creation and consolidation of a welfare state, changed the role and functions of the British state (e.g. Crosland, 1956; Hayek, 1976; Jessop, 1980; Sullivan 1987; Taylor-Gooby, 1991).

What is often at issue is the nature of this transformation. Each of the perspectives on the state considered in this chapter theorises the nature in different ways. The social democratic perspective adopted by revisionist writers, sees this as more fundamental than any of the other perspectives, save that from the radical right. This sees the transformation of the state in the late 1940s as the natural conclusion of the capitalist system itself:

> While capitalism has not collapsed as a result of internal contradictions – it is possible to see a transformation of capitalism occurring. Since 1945 capitalism has been undergoing a metamorphosis into a different system. (Crosland, 1952, p. 34)

or, in Crossman's words, 'capitalism had been civilised'.

This transformation of capitalism rested on a number of factors. Crosland (1952) provides the clearest account of the process and reasons for this supposed capitalist transformation. First, the growth of powerful anti-capitalist movements (the Labour Party, trade unions, etc.) during the early twentieth century had led to the formation of a reform coalition whose aspirations for a changed society could not be ignored by Conservative or radical governments. Second, it is argued, the British business class also supported the political aspirations of the labour movement, though for different reasons, and therefore supported the transformation of the state into an interventionist state. Here the major political impulse arose from an analysis that large scale state intervention policies benefited capital as well as labour. Full employment (one of the identifiers of the interventionist state) meant guaranteed high levels of consumption and production, which in turn meant high profit levels for producers. Further, it is asserted that the inter-war recession had led many owners and managers of capital to question the efficacy, and perhaps even the morality, of unbridled capitalism. As a consequence, British capitalists had developed something approaching a social conscience, and conscience and self-interest became comfortable bedfellows.

Transformation of the state, and particularly the commitment to full employment and state welfare state services, therefore occurred with the support or acquiescence of the capitalist class itself. Fourth, the dispersion of ownership and increasing control of industry by a managerial class had led, according to Crosland, to the transformation of capitalism as an economic system. Exploitative, entrepreneurial capitalism had evolved to give birth to a system under which ownership and power had been dispersed and exploitation diminished. Finally, according to this revisionist thesis, the level of state planning developed during the Second World War had made a return to free-market capitalism impossible. As far as the revisionist thinkers were concerned, capitalism had spawned a new economic and social system. This metamorphosis amounted to no less than the adoption by the state of regulation of social and economic relationships in British society – a role previously occupied largely by the market.

This theme is also developed by T. H. Marshall in his work on citizenship and social class (1963, 1971). For Marshall, the transmutation of capitalism was the result of a cumulative process in which a new consensus within British society had been forged over time. The agreements related to the legal, political and social rights which citizens should enjoy in a capitalist state. With the arrival of state welfare in the twentieth century, a complete package of citizen rights had been integrated into the capitalist system. This package regulated capitalism and protected individuals from the ravages of unbridled market forces. In so doing, capitalism had, itself, spawned a new set of economic and social institutions that had altered its very nature (Marshall, 1963).

The source of state authority

Implicit in the above discussion is the view that the new, transformed and interventionist state drew its authority and legitimacy
from a societal consensus that had been forged around a new understanding of the relationship between state and civil society. That
such a consensus could be fashioned was itself evidence of the evolution of the capitalist system. Important elements in the creation of
this new consensus included, as we have seen, the growth of a countervailing power bloc (the trade union and labour movement) and
its ability to compete with the power of owners of industrial capital:
changes in the ownership and control structure of capitalism itself;
and a realisation by the representatives of industrial capital that a
state that guaranteed full employment also guaranteed high profits.

It would be a mistake, however, to underestimate the importance
that this perspective accords to the growth of social conscience as a
component in creating and moulding a new consensus. The interventionist state is seen as legitimised not only by a new accommodation to political and economic realities but also by the growth of a
collective conscience, seen as based on rational/moral calculus.
From this perspective, the powerful (the capitalist or business class),
having witnessed at first hand the privations of the powerless (the
workers, or more accurately workless caused by prolonged economic recession), formed part of a moral and rational consensus on the
need for state regulation and intervention. Such intervention would
ameliorate or prevent such conditions occurring in the future. As we
shall see (Chapter 4), such an analysis forms an important strand in
social democratic perspectives on state intervention in welfare.

The source of authority and legitimation for increased state activity in the post-war years is seen, then, as rooted in a groundswell
of interest and opinion hostile to, or at least critical of, the results
of unchecked capitalism. Continued legitimation of state activity
would depend on a continued social consensus in favour of intervention, but the revisionists had little doubt of the stability and
endurance of that consensus.

The state and government

As we shall see later, the relationship between the state and
government is, particularly in Marxist perspectives, theoretically

problematic. For the revisionists no such problem arises. The state, or the apparatus of government, is seen as subordinate to the will of democratically elected governments. The policies and actions of the state are no more and no less than the policies of elected governments. The policies and actions of governments are, themselves, simply responses to a societal consensus (however forged) on the nature of government policies. Illustrations of this approach litter the literature of social democracy but it is nowhere more clearly stated than in an essay by Strachey in Crossman's collection of Fabian essays (Crossman, 1952). Commenting on what he regarded as the formation of a socialist consensus in Britain in the late 1940s, Strachey argues in the same breath for two revisionist propositions: that the state is subordinate to government and that capitalism has been transformed by state interventionist measures. 'Keynesian fiscal measures supplemented by physical controls gave the state all the tools that were needed to enable it to do what it wanted' (Strachey, in Crossman, 1952, p. 188).

For Strachey there is no question that the state machinery was subordinate to the will of government. A new consensus, expressed through government policies, had meant that the early post-war period was characterised by 'governments accepting as state responsibility what had previously been left to the free market' (Crosland, 1956, p. 11). According to social democratic theories, the state, though autonomous from the owners of capital, possessed no autonomy from government. It was no more and no less than its handmaiden. Such a view had been clearly expressed by Labour's first post-war Prime Minister, reflecting on the relationship between government and civil service 'that's the civil service tradition, a great tradition. They carry out the policy of any given government' (Williams, 1969, p. 79).

For the revisionists, then, the state, operating within the context of a transformed capitalism, occupied a handmaiden role to government. That state had been used by governments following the Second World War, to encourage and legitimise the metamorphosis of dominant values in British society from the values of competitive capitalism to values of co-operation and collectivism (Tawney, 1964, p. 169).

The role and functions of the state

Already it has been argued that from the social democratic view the state occupies a subservient role to that of government and acts simply to implement government policy. In particular the state, as the instrument of government, functions to regulate and iron out peripheral problems in a reasonably harmonious and humane social system. It also functions to lay down the ground rules that would ensure the consolidation and development of the social democratic consensus that had emerged in the post-war period. Specifically the roles of the British state are, in this social democratic formulation, threefold.

1. 'The state acts to correct, supplement and, if necessary, supplant the market system to promote the development of greater equality, democracy and welfare in British society' (George and Wilding, 1985). It was, after all, clear to the social democrats that, in a liberal-democratic, mixed economy society with a plurality of power bases and economic control, the state would sometimes have to operate to lay down the detailed ground rules and compel the private (and nationalised) corporation to conform to its own views of where the public interest lies (Crosland, 1974) or to guide the private (and public) sector to forms of collective action to achieve collective goals which individuals cannot achieve, or cannot achieve with the same measure of success, by their isolated efforts (Crosland, 1956).

2. 'The social democratic state operates to modify injustices caused by a market system of resource distribution' (George and Wilding, 1985). Even in a post-war Britain characterised by the emergence of a new social consensus, the private sector of the economy was seen to be motivated by profit rather than the desire to satisfy social and economic needs. The state, in such a system, would operate – largely by means of social expenditure – to redistribute resources, whether through the tax and income maintenance systems or through services in kind.

3. The social democratic state operates to develop a planned growth economy in order to facilitate redistributive social and economic policies. If the diminution of inequalities was an important goal for the revisionist socialists then it was seen as imperative that the state should act as a planning agency operating to develop Britain into a continuous growth economy generating wealth to be used for redistributive purposes.

For the revisionists then, the state has clear functions to perform. They are underwritten by government and rooted in a social consensus on the goals of state action. To perform those functions and achieve consensual goals, the state would therefore act, particularly through Keynesian economic measures (Schott, 1982), to stimulate and guide the economy, and through social welfare measures to ensure continued consensus.

In other words, according to this perspective, the state is and should be used as an agency of economic planning, regulation and reorganisation to maintain full employment in the British economy. Full employment, it is argued, generates high production levels and additional national wealth. These, in turn, generate higher levels of social expenditure as well as promoting higher levels of consumption.

The state, in this perspective, also acts through a strategy of increased social expenditure to ameliorate residual relative deprivation and to redistribute resources. It should be stressed that this perspective neither promotes, nor prescribes the eradication of inequality as a state function. Rather, it sees the state operating to modify the scope of inequalities between individuals. The provision of a welfare minimum is seen, in this perspective, as having two related aims. The first is to ameliorate and modify resource inequalities but the second, and arguably more important, is to guarantee an equality of status – rather than outcome – to all citizens through access to state welfare services (Crosland, 1956; Marshall, 1963).

Understanding state activity in post-war Britain

How, then, does this perspective on the state help us to understand patterns of state involvement in post-war British economic and social life?

As we have seen, large scale intervention in both economy and social policy during the three decades of interventionism is easily explained by the social democrats. A new social consensus had been forged during the war and post-war years around a growth economy consisting of public and private sectors. This full employment growth economy was achieved largely as a result of state interventionist Keynesian policies of planning, stimulation and

But blown away by [...]

industrial reorganisation. The post-war consensus also embraced the idea of using economic growth and national prosperity to enhance social expenditure and provide increased citizen access to welfare services.

During this period, the state, as a tool of government, was increasingly interventionist. Its activities were marked by expansion and continuity whichever political party was in government. This, then, constituted the orthodox post-war view of the role, functions and legitimacy of the British state. Or it did so until the oil-shocks of the 1970s. Challenges to this orthodoxy were to emerge and were to be generated by ideological and fiscal disputes. In part, these challenges were simply developments of existing critiques of the mixed economy welfare state. In the 1980s and 1990s, as in earlier decades, social democratic understandings were, as we shall see, attacked by a pincer movement from the political left and the political right. By the 1980s, however, these hitherto marginal analyses had become more clearly enunciated and, to some at least, more persuasive. Before looking at the apparent eclipse of social democratic values and the renaissance of critical views from the right and left in the recent period, some time needs to be spent scrutinising the bases of these critiques.

Marxist views of the state

More extensive, detailed and sophisticated summaries of Marxist theories of the state exist than the one that follows (Gold *et al.*, 1975; Jessop, 1977). Readers will also find in the extensive corpus of work (Miliband, 1969, 1982; Poulantzas, 1972, 1975; Jessop, 1977, 1980) much richer accounts of the diverse analyses, controversies and debates within Marxist scholarship about the nature, role and functions of the capitalist state. The aim here is to present an account of those elements of Marxist scholarship that help us begin to make sense of the development of state social and economic intervention in modern Britain viewed from outside social democracy.

An ambiguity or duality about the nature of the state in capitalist society appears to exist in the writings of Marx himself. On the one hand, he appears to argue that the state is no more and no less than the organising committee of a ruling or capitalist class that always acts to promote, foster and protect the economic cultural and ideological interests of that class (Marx, 1967). However, in other places he appears to argue that the state has a degree of autonomy from society in general and from a ruling class or elite in particular. In the 'Eighteenth Brumaire', for example, he appears to suggest that the state does not merely co-ordinate society in the interests of a ruling class. Rather, it can in particular circumstances – especially when there is a relative balance of social class forces – promote changes and developments in civil society that are not immediately recognisable as actions in the interest of a dominant class (Marx, 1973). What follows, therefore, is an attempt to describe how this duality is reflected in Marxist writing on the state. Two approaches – which may be described as system determinist (or Marxist functionalist) and relative autonomy approaches – are traced to see what they have to say about the activities and nature of the state in society.

A transformed state

The social democratic view depends on the idea of a transformed state to explain post-war developments. Marxist theories of the state also rely, in part, on the idea of state transformation. For some writers, changes in the activities of the state imply accommodating modifications in the nature of capitalism over time. They amount to little more than historically specific strategies to promote the interests of a dominant class. Thus, if the state in twentieth-century capitalist countries intervenes in the economy to stabilise demand for industrial products in a way hitherto unknown, there is a straightforward explanation for such activity. Entrepreneurial capitalism has been replaced during the present century by corporate capitalism; the greater complexity of corporate capitalism and its greater distance from the market for its products demand state intervention (Baran and Sweezy, 1968; Mandel, 1968).

Similarly, if the state in modern times has intervened in welfare to a far greater extent than hitherto, then such intervention, and the transformation of state activities that it betokens, are again merely historically specific strategies to protect the interests of a capitalist class. Welfare interventions may have been introduced to ensure stability of consumption for corporate capitalism (Mandel, 1968), to provide an appropriately socialised, educated and healthy workforce for capitalist enterprise (Saville, 1957; O'Connor, 1973), or to supplement the repressive and ideological state apparatuses with a conformative element (Barratt-Brown, 1972). State transformations are, from a system determinist Marxist approach, more illusory than real.

Other Marxist writers, however, accord greater significance to transformations in state activity. Jessop, commenting on the fundamental changes in state activity in the early post-war period, is in little doubt that 'this produced a major transformation of the British state and implied a fundamental social democratisation of the political system' (Scase, 1980, p. 27). Post-war policy interventions by the state are similarly seen by other writers as reflecting real rather than illusory transformations in the relationship between state, society and social classes, whether temporary or permanent. For some, such transformations reflect limited autonomy for the state from a ruling class (Miliband, 1969); for others they reflect a much greater degree of autonomy through which the interests of all members of society are expressed via the workings of the capitalist state (Offe and Ronge, 1975).

As we see later in this chapter, these differences in emphasis imply quite different analyses of the role and functions of the capitalist state as well as of the sources of its legitimacy.

The source of state authority

Whereas the social democratic perspective sees society as characterised by a broad consensus on values, goals and interests, of which state action is merely a reflection, Marxist theories of the state are rooted in analyses that see society as characterised by value, goal and interest conflict. Such conflicts are considered to be components of the fundamental clash between a dominant or ruling class and a subordinate or working class. However, this view of society yields somewhat different analyses of the sources of state authority according to the sorts of Marxists.

Put simply, a system determinist view sees the ultimate authority for state intervention in civil society as being the interests of a dominant social class. That class may seek through some, or all, of those state actions to legitimise its interests by presenting class interests as national or universal interests (George and Wilding, 1976, 1985). However, final authority for state action lies in promoting ruling class interests, whether through actions aimed at creating the conditions for optimum capital accumulation or through interventions aimed at legitimising that process (O'Connor, 1973).

Relative autonomy approaches permit the interpretation that the authority and legitimacy of the state (and of state interventions) rest in the theoretical or actual possibility of the state acting in the interests of a wider constituency than that represented by a dominant social class. That autonomy may be restricted to acting, at times, against certain sections of the dominant class (Poulantzas, 1973, 1975), or may be extensive enough to allow representation of apparently conflicting interests (Ginsburg, 1979; Gough, 1979). None the less, for relative autonomists the source of authority for state activity and the legitimacy of state intervention is built on a more extensive foundation than that erected by system determinists.

The state and government

Whereas social democratic writers perceive an unproblematic relationship between state and government, and see the former as being the instrument of the latter, Marxist writers see the relationship as a complex one. Marxists, whether of the system determinist or relative autonomy brand, are united in their agreement on the following:

1. The state is to a greater or lesser extent generally predisposed to act in the long term interests of a dominant class in society. This may be because of the social provenance of senior state personnel (instrumental theories of the state, Miliband, 1969, 1978, 1982). It may be the result of a class structure that ensures ruling class dominance of the state whatever the social provenance of its personnel (structuralist theories of the state, Poulantzas, 1973, 1975).
2. Such a state will therefore tend to act as a conservative force, at least for much of the time.

r the possibilities of state autonomy from a dominant
most of the time the state will act as a conservative
ιᴏιᴄᴄ wiiatever the political complexion of government.

In general, therefore, the state will occupy, at best, a semi-autonomous relationship to government. Certainly, during the occupancy of reforming governments, the state may not act as the subordinate instrument of government implementing policy made by government but may act as an alternative, and generally more powerful, centre of policy-making. In theory, the state will manifest a similar relative autonomy from government, even when government is itself conservative in nature. Such an analysis led Marxists in two different directions. System determinists generally argued that, as a consequence of this analysis, the only route to social change is one predicated on destroying the capitalist state (Mandel, 1968). Relative autonomy writers, on the other hand, argued that such an analysis points to the further need to transform the state by taking control of it.

The role and functions of the state

The foregoing discussion will have made it patently clear that, for the system determinists at least, the post-war state occupied a handmaiden role to the interests of capitalism and of a dominant, ruling class or elite. For them the state, in its interventionist activities, acted to protect, reinforce and reproduce the economic, social and political relationships of capitalist society (Barratt-Brown, 1972). Most importantly, it acted through economic intervention to promote capital accumulation (O'Connor, 1973) or economic efficiency (Saville, 1957). It also operated through social intervention (the provision of welfare) to accord citizens a modicum of social rights which often aided the accumulation process. Such interventions may be regarded as activities intended to legitimise the relationships of capitalist society (O'Connor, 1973) or, in other analyses, as conformative activities (Barratt-Brown, 1972). As a result, welfare and similar state institutions and activities have been regarded as ideological state apparatuses (Althusser, 1971).

From this viewpoint, the state is also seen as acting coercively, especially during periods when the state's legitimising or conformative activities have failed to ensure adequate levels of conformity to the values and relationships of capitalism. It may do so to ensure social stability – one of capitalism's prime requisites (Saville, 1957). This role involves, naturally enough, the legal, law enforcement and security services of the state, Althusser's repressive state apparatuses (Althusser, 1971).

Thus, the state:

> by its very nature . . . is simply coercive power used to protect the system of rights and duties of one process of economic relationships from invasion by another class which seeks to change them in the interest of another process. (Laski, 1934, p. 118)

In contrast, a somewhat different picture emerges from the work of those writers who theorise the existence of a degree of relative autonomy for the state from the interests of capitalism and a ruling class. Relative autonomy theories of the state present a wide range of views on the role and functions of the state in post-war capitalist society.

Poulantzas (1973, 1975), arguing that the capitalist class is less homogeneous than system determinist approaches allow, sees the dominant class as composed of class fractions (industrial capital, finance capital, etc.) which may, from time to time, have different and competing interests. He develops a model of the state that is relatively autonomous from each and all of these class fractions, but which acts in the long-term interests of capitalism. It does so by performing functions and activities that protect the long-term survival interests of capitalism as a system. The state, therefore, adopts a semi-autonomous role in relation to the different sectors of the capitalist class but functions to perpetuate the capitalist class system.

Other writers see the post-war state as predisposed to adopt a supportive role to the capitalist system but which functions in a secondary and contingent way to promote some of the interests of subordinate social classes:

> From the working class view, it is a response to their continual struggle . . . . From the capitalist point of view it has contributed to the continual struggle to accumulate capital . . . in bringing labour and capital together profitably. (Ginsburg, 1979, p. 2)

Still others (Gough, 1979, for instance) see the post-war state's relative autonomy as manifest especially during periods of approximate balance in the social class struggle. At such times the state may act to promote interests that are not those of a dominant class and its role may therefore be seen as one of representing majority interests in society (Offe and Ronge, 1975).

Yet another strand in this relative autonomy thesis points up state activities that appear to reflect a coincidental coalition of interests between social classes at particular times. Such a strand comes near to presenting the state as capable, at particular historical points, of reflecting and moulding a national or supra-class interest (see Bellaby, 1977, for instance).

The role and functions of the state in capitalist society are thus seen from a somewhat different perspective by system determinists, on the one hand, and by relative autonomy writers on the other. Such differences stem from different concepts of the relationship between the state and social class(es), and are also reflected in the different ways in which they seek to explain state intervention in British society in the post-war period.

Understanding state activity in post-war Britain

Marxist explanations of state activity in post-war Britain provide a rich, complex and diverse set of accounts for state interventionism (Saville, 1957; Baran and Sweezy, 1968; Mandel, 1968; Offe and Ronge, 1975; Gough, 1979; Offe, 1984). While system determinist writers tend to perceive state interventionist policies as performing functional tasks aimed at perpetuating a capitalist system of social organisation, Marxist writers concede the existence of a less deterministic relationship between state activity and capitalist interests.

For the system determinists there is an almost inevitable relationship between the interests of a capitalist class and the activities of the state. Thus the Keynesian economic strategy of demand management adopted in the early post-war years may be seen as little more than state activity designed to promote the interests of the owners of capital in British society (Baran and Sweezy, 1968). Planned full employment in a controlled economy stimulated demand and consumption, and contributed to a process of capital accumulation. In a slightly weaker variant of the system determinist line, intervention in economy and industry – although a concession to an ascendant subject class – was planned and implemented in such a way that the economic interests of a capitalist class would not be damaged, and may indeed have been improved (Schott, 1982).

The large scale intervention of the state in social policy through the creation and consolidation of a welfare state may, from this approach, also be seen as part of a strategy aimed at protecting and promoting the interests of capital. So that the creation of a national health service might be seen as promoting the economic interests of capitalism by maintaining the health of workers and potential workers. Education provision might be seen as promoting both economic and ideological interests by functioning to produce appropriately skilled and appropriately socialised workers, and so on (see Chapter 4 for a further treatment of these issues).

State intervention to reorganise or reorient industry in the 1960s, together with specific welfare interventions in education and income maintenance, can be seen, through the eyes of the system determinists, as providing further evidence that state intervention in civil society functions to protect, promote and reinforce capitalist interests.

The expansion of higher education with an accompanying emphasis on technology, together with the reorganisation of secondary education, took place at a time when the state was also increasing its interventionist powers to modernise industry and facilitate technological development. Each of these initiatives might be seen as part of an interventionist package to increase Britain's industrial competitiveness and promote quicker economic growth which, in turn, would contribute to increased levels of profit for the owners of capital. The introduction of a new element in the income maintenance system, namely, an earnings related unemployment benefit offering reasonably high levels of benefit to the frictionally unemployed, might be seen as a welfare intervention aimed at minimising the opposition of labour organisations to such economic and industrial restructuring.

The picture that emerges, then, is of an interventionist state operating at least until the end of the 1960s, in a way that, while maintaining full employment and providing extensive welfare services, ultimately served the interests of a dominant social class. This analysis was further developed during the late 1970s and early 1980s. What emerged from Marxism's attempt to grapple with the early experiments in neo-liberal economics and radical right ideology is discussed below.

Marxism and the state: the oil-shock economy

During the earliest post-war period, the process of capital accumulation had been aided by the activities of an interventionist state operating a demand management economic strategy. Economic planning, a strategy of full employment and welfare interventions had together formed the basis for economic growth and protection of the economic interests of a dominant class. However, by the early 1970s Keynesianism was in crisis. The British economy – whose growth had, in any case, been slower than both that planned and that of its competitors – was faltering. Unemployment was rising. In such a situation, a comprehensive system of welfare services and high levels of public spending which had hitherto complemented capital accumulation, now had the opposite effect. High levels of public expenditure, taking up an ever-increasing proportion of gross national product, threatened capital accumulation rather than aiding it (O'Connor, 1973). In these new circumstances, this contradiction of capitalism – as it was seen – was best resolved by state activity aimed at reducing public expenditure, and therefore reducing state intervention in some areas. This was particularly so in those areas appropriately resourced in a growth economy – for example, education and health – but inappropriate to the needs of a contracting economy with a slack labour market. Important elements of state interventionist powers, especially in economic and industrial planning and control, were retained by governments anticipating the deepening recession to be but part of a cyclical process of slump and boom. Most notably, both sides of industry were incorporated, at least partially, into the machinery of the state in an attempt to manage the recession by consent.

With the deepening economic crisis in Britain during the late 1970s and early 1980s, came new patterns of state activity aimed at shoring up and, if possible, improving the prospects of the owners of capital. The state, acting as the 'politically conscious directorate' of capital and aided by a new Conservative government substantially shorn of adherence to the aristocratic paternalism of previous Conservative governments, set about steering a new course.

The contradictory nature of state involvement in the 1970s had failed to halt economic decline. Public spending restrictions co-ordinated by a corporate state had failed woefully to stanch Britain's economic wounds. Capitalism and state involvement were therefore to move into a stage with new guiding principles. They were to be

1. Rolling back the state from large scale expenditure and involvement in the public sector of industry and the public services (including welfare). This dismantling of the interventionist state would allow market forces to reassert themselves as the guiding hand of the economy. Such a free market, released from the burden of financing public enterprises and services, would reverse Britain's economic fortunes and lead to a growth in profitability.
2. A specific intention to dismantle the welfare state: its support functions were, after all, unnecessary in a possibly permanent period of high unemployment. Individual family and community 'needs' for welfare should be met, wherever possible by individuals, families and communities. The legitimation of dominant values previously facilitated by elements of the Welfare State (e.g. education and personal social services) would, less expensively, be achieved by coercive means.
3. The removal of controls on the export of capital, which would facilitate capital accumulation by permitting investment in high profit economies such as those in the Far East.

As we have seen in Chapter 2, such a strategy for state activity in the 1980s has thrown up a number of paradoxes or contradictions. That the rhetoric and reality of rolling back the state do not completely match each other is indisputable. High levels of unemployment have meant increased public spending on income maintenance provisions. The failure of insurance schemes for health and education in other societies has, perhaps, inhibited the privatisation of welfare services, though it has not prevented restrictions in spending. It may even be that public resistance has obstructed a more rapid and substantial removal of the state from the arena of civil society.

Marxists who adopt a system determinist approach must conceptualise such difficulties as pointing up the contradictions capitalism has created for itself rather than as in any part reflecting a political

et resolved. The state is experiencing temporary diffi-
ioving itself from crucial areas of social and economic
ifficulties are accompanied, as we have seen, by a need
to sur...g n the state in some other areas. Such contradictions
demonstrate contemporary problems in representing the interest
of a social class of which the state is a creature. They do not and
cannot illustrate that the British state in the 1980s, as in other
periods, was caught in a tension between two sets of conflicting
interests, neither of which it fully represents.

Those writing from a less determinist Marxist position appear to
understand state activity in the post-war period somewhat dif-
ferently. According to some (Miliband, 1969, 1978, 1982), the state
has, during this period, seldom acted to promote the interests of
sections of the population other than a dominant elite or class.
This is largely so because of the similarity in social provenance and
social values between that dominant elite and senior state functionaries. None the less, the state is seen, at least theoretically, as
an arena for struggle capable of transformation by replacing its
functionaries and, consequently, their interests and values.

Others see certain interventions by the state during the period, as
having actually reflected the interests of a much wider constituency
than a small elite. The creation and early consolidation of the welfare state may be seen as an example of such interventions reflecting
the state's relative autonomy and capacity to act on behalf of wider
interests, especially at times when the balance of power between
social classes in society is more evenly poised than at others (Gough,
1979). Some proponents of this approach would also wish to explain
some interventionist developments as truly reflecting the dialectical
nature of class struggle. To take but two examples, the reorganisation of secondary education (Bellaby, 1977) and the expansion of
higher education may be seen as activities yielding advantages to
competing social class interests while failing to satisfy the total demands of either. Thus the provision of secondary and higher education, ostensibly aimed at producing equality of opportunity to
students from different social classes, may be seen as partially reflecting that aspiration as well as producing appropriately educated
and socialised person power for capitalist enterprise.

The ultimate failure of Keynesianism in the 1970s and the overload of government (O'Connor, 1973) threw organised labour on
to the defensive and in such circumstances, the state more clearly

acted in the interests of a ruling elite. None the less, the failure of the Thatcher governments to fully implement policies of state retrenchment should be seen, in part, as a response to growing resistance to such retrenchment from wider sections of the population (Taylor-Gooby, 1985; Papadakis and Taylor-Gooby, 1987; Sullivan, 1992).

Radical right views on the state

Even the most cursory of reading of the 'giants' of the radical right (Hayek, 1944, 1949, 1960, 1973, 1979; Friedman, 1962; Friedman and Friedman, 1980), or indeed, of their contemporary British disciples (Seldon, 1967, 1981; Powell, 1969; Boyson, 1971; Harris and Seldon, 1979, 1987; Joseph and Sumption, 1979; Minford, 1984; Gilder, 1988; Katz, 1989; Murray, 1990) leaves the reader in no doubt that for the writers and actors of the radical right, extensive state activity in civil society over the post-war period is to be regretted. It has translated aspirations into citizen rights (Powell, 1972, p. 12). It has overturned a free-market system that acted as a guarantor of individual freedom. The interventionist state has substantially transformed an earlier form of social organisation, in which political power was held by one group and economic power by a countervailing force that could use its power to block state coercion (Friedman, 1962). It has created business and labour monopolies that limit voluntary exchange. It has fostered waste and inefficiency, and reduced the population to the status of serfdom (Hayek, 1944).

For the radical right, analysis of the state was, at least for the first thirty or so welfare state years, a straightforward process. This, as we have seen, was the period of social democratic hegemony. The critique of social democratisation of the state constructed by the right over this stretch of time was, therefore, a commentary from the vantage point of political opposition. It was not until the last years of the 1970s that the conceptual road map developed by these thinkers was put to the service of political activists negotiating the route of political, economic and social change. As we shall see later, this new task generated clearer prescriptions for action than the critique of orthodox state interventionism developed in the earlier welfare state period.

A transformed state

Radical right commentators were quite clear that the increased involvement of the state in the affairs of civil society since 1945 marks a transformation in the nature of the state. That transformation is perceived, by many, as having been from a minimalist state with residual economic and social functions to a collectivist state with extensive central planning functions in the economy and welfare (Hayek, 1960; Harris and Seldon, 1979). More sharply, the transformation is seen by some as having replaced a liberal non-interventionist state with an embryonic socialist state conducive to the development of an authoritarian society (e.g. Powell, 1969).

The source of state authority

As we have seen already, different perspectives on the state offer quite different analyses of the processes which legitimise interventionist state activity. From the social democratic viewpoint, the source of state authority is seen as being rooted in a societal consensus on the need for an interventionist state which functions to transform, or humanise, the capitalist system. For Marxists writing from a system determinist standpoint, the logic of capitalism – and particularly of capital accumulation – acts as the source of legitimation for state activity. For relative autonomy writers, state activities are legitimised because the state is an arena of struggle theoretically, and sometimes actually, capable of representing the interest of a wider constituency than a ruling class or elite.

For writers from the radical right, none of these understandings will suffice. Rather the state, in its interventionist activities, drew support from a social consensus created through a process of misapprehension. For these writers the interventionist state was a half-way house to socialism or, indeed, 'socialism by stealth' (Powell, 1969). The British population had been misled by well-meaning but mistaken reformers who drew the British public and state along the road to collectivism and created a semi-authoritarian state and a subject, fettered people (Hayek, 1944; Friedman and Friedman, 1980). Put quite simply, the state's authority for interventionist actions was seen as bogus, rooted in the creation of a false consensus based on false premises and was the subject of close scrutiny.

The state and government

Radical right views of the relationship between state and government are very interesting. It should be clear by now that the ultimate aim of the radical right thinkers in the pre-Thatcher era was the creation of a society stripped of state interventionism except in those few areas where market regulation and provision is inappropriate or inefficient (Boyson, 1971; Harris and Seldon, 1979; Seldon 1981). Radical right views of this period on what constituted authority to roll back the state, provide an interesting insight into how the relationship between government and state is theorised in new right thought. It has been a central argument by proponents of this view that the sole authority for a minimalist state would be that gained through an electoral mandate. This mirrors, of course, the view from the right that the source of authority for post-war state interventionism was a societal consensus, albeit based on a form of false consciousness (Powell, 1972). What emerges, therefore is a view that the level of state activity in society has been and can be regulated by the political will of societal members. That political will, however formed, is reflected in support for a particular political party as government and that government, once elected, occupies a superordinate position to the state. In this respect at least, writers of the new right have a notion of the state which is surprisingly close to that of social democratic writers.

The role and functions of the state

For much of the post-war period the state has, from this perspective, played a role which, despite the legitimacy ascribed by societal consensus, promoted the interests of collectivism and collective planning, and repressed the interests of individual freedom and democracy. Specifically the state, as a result of its interventionist activities, operated in such a way that the fabric of a civilised society and healthy economy was threatened. For the anti-collectivist writers of the new right, post-war collectivist and interventionist state activities were socially disruptive, reduced freedom, wasted resources and promoted economic inefficiency (George and Wilding, 1976, 1985). State interventionism, particularly in social policy, raised expectations, through a theory of universal services, that individual *needs* should be treated as individual *rights*. It conspired to disappoint these expectations for a variety of reasons – detailed in Chapter 4 – and therefore acted as a disruptive force in British society. State provision of services in many areas created virtual monopolies, with the resultant effects of limiting individual freedom of choice in the consumption of services (Powell, 1972) and wasting resources because of the removal of competition.

In contrast to this, the radical right argued, the state should be substantially withdrawn from essentially political activities. It should perform only residual economic/social functions in a society reformed to permit maximum individual freedom and minimum state interference. In such a society economic efficiency and growth as well as individual choice are promoted by the mechanisms of a free market. The state's functions in such a society are limited to those areas which 'cannot be handled through the market at all, or can be handled at so great a cost that the use of political channels may be preferable' (Friedman, 1962, p. 25). Such functions might include:

(a) a rule-making and arbitration function and in particular the administration of legal and justice systems;
(b) a function to provide services where state monopoly is likely to be more technically efficient than competitive non-state provision (perhaps rail services and the like); and
(c) a function to provide services and design policies for individuals no longer capable of making informed individual choices (such as the mentally ill and the mentally handicapped) (George and Wilding, 1976).

Such an understanding of post-war state functions is reflected in the following discussion of the post-war British state.

Understanding state activity in post-war Britain

Here, as elsewhere in the writings of the new right, explanations are deceptively simple. If we are to understand the large scale interventionist activities of the state during the three decades of interventionism, we only have to understand one thing. Successive governments, as well as generations of British people, fell prey to the 'false trails of Butskellism', to a vision of planned economy (albeit a mixed economy), full employment and rights to welfare. They were misled, and misled themselves, into believing that central state intervention could create a just, humane and efficient society. In so doing, governments as well as people, while rejecting the ends of authoritarian socialism, embraced the means of achieving those ends.

That such a process was reversed, or at least inhibited from the mid-1970s on, was the result of a number of factors. Chief among them however, were the following:

1. The interventionist state failed to achieve the aims set for it, whether for sustained economic growth or for the provision of universal, non-stigmatising welfare services. Such failures perceived by people and governments threw seriously into question the hope that state interventionism could ever fulfil its promise (see Sullivan, 1989).
2. There was the effect of government overload. Throughout the three decades following 1945, successive governments had increased levels of state intervention in British society. By the mid-1970s it had become crystal clear that, with the failure of Keynesian economic policies to generate domestic economic growth and with the economic storm clouds gathering over the world economy, state activities of the scope already existing could no longer be financed.

Such logic became apparent to the Labour government of the mid-1970s and led to certain limited, if significant, changes in state expenditure. State interventionist social and economic policies therefore became, in the late 1970s, sandwiched between the rock of fiscal crisis and the hard place of a legitimation crisis, in part created by the apparent inability of social democracy to understand and cope with economic crisis and government overload.

The hegemony of social democratic notions of state action came under severe threat even before Callaghan's buffeted Labour government fell in 1979. Though, as we shall see later, the Conservative party garnered the major political advantage from the collapse of reformism, the seeds of collapse had been identified by some post-war Marxist writers (see especially, O'Connor, 1973). They drew attention to the inherent fragility of the post-war settlement

(Mandel, 1968; O'Connor, 1973). For them, capitalism coexisted with collectivist politics only as a means of protecting itself in particular historical circumstances. Once those circumstances altered, the ideological compact between capital and labour would founder under the weight of fiscal and doctrinal attack. Though ordinary citizens may have benefited, alongside capitalism, from the growth of citizen rights to economic security and welfare, the ballast of the mixed economy welfare state settlement had been capital's willingness to administer welfare capitalism. By the late 1970s that ballast was being removed.

Ideas about the state in the 1980s and 1990s

The election in 1979 of a Conservative government headed by Mrs Margaret Thatcher marked the beginning of significant changes in state action. The remodelling of state action in social policy is detailed in Chapter 4. What is of interest here are ideas about the nature of the state which have developed following the collapse of social democratic theories.

The minimalist state

As is clear elsewhere (Riddell, 1983; Sullivan, 1987, 1989, 1992; Young, 1989), ideas of a minimalist state dominated early post-consensus political discussions. Traditional radical right thinking pointed to the distortions created by the social democratic state and prescribed its demise (Hayek, 1944, 1960; Friedman and Friedman, 1980; Harris and Seldon, 1979). Other developments outside the United Kingdom also influenced the way in which new right thinkers and new Conservative politicians thought about the state. Chief among these influences was the election of an unreconstructed economic neo-liberal to the United States Presidency. Reagan's ideology and his actions, both of which influenced the British Prime Minister, emphasised the removal of the state from activities which could be provided efficiently by the private sector. Similarly, in the United Kingdom, there was much support for 'rolling back the state', especially during the early 1980s. Policies emanating from this approach to the state included innovations in industrial policy and in social policy. Previously nationalised industries were to be returned to the private sector. This would allow the entrepreneurial skills of private corporations to develop more efficient and more profitable services and would remove a financial burden (or bonus) from the shoulders of the state and the taxpayer. State welfare monopolies were to be challenged by private competitors or, as seemed likely in the case of the NHS from 1979 to 1982, abolished and replaced by some private means of provision.

State and government were to be pruned. Big government was bad government. The state would be left only with those activities that it could address more efficiently and more effectively than non-state agencies.

The enabling state

Over time, ideas about the removal of the state gave way to another political formulation on the appropriate role of the state in civil society. This new idea saw the retention of the state in many of those areas where it had previously been active. The role of state agencies was, however, to change. No longer would the tentacles of the state stretch into the lives of each and every person through its administration of economic, industrial and social policy. Instead, the state should adopt an *enabling role*. This change of perception on the radical right, or at least among new Conservative political practitioners, dating from about 1983, was intended to cater not only for the failure of the first Thatcher government to roll back the state (see Chapters 1 and 4) but also to give practical expression to a post-social democratic concept of the state. In this notion, state agencies which had previously been responsible for the provision of some sort of service were to be transformed into enablers or commissioners of service. This idea and its implications is considered in depth when we look at approaches to social policy later. Suffice to say here, that many recent government initiatives have the idea of the enabling state at their core.

Conclusion

For much of the post-war period, then, a social democratic idea of the appropriate relationship between state and civil society held sway. Though dominant, it and the political actions that stemmed from it, found critics to the left and right of social democracy. While Marxism mounted a critique of the idea of a beneficent and neutral state, radical rightism regretted the use of the state to create and nurture collectivist politics. The crisis for social democracy came in the years following global oil shocks in the mid-1970s. Caught between fiscal and legitimation crises, social democratic theory and action appeared bankrupt. Though Marxist analyses of the fragility of post-war settlement now seemed warranted, it was the resurgent right that moved to the centre of the political stage, and it is their ideas about the state that have formed the political currency of the last two decades.

CHAPTER 4

Understanding welfare

Pre-Thatcherite social policy

Chapter 3 was primarily concerned with a range of ideas about state intervention in the social and economic organisation of post-war British society. The views considered there yielded significantly different interpretations of the nature, role and functions of the contemporary British state. In consequence, they also yielded different understandings of state activities in post-war Britain.

The aim of this chapter and the next is to understand the changes in modern social policy and in state involvement with the provision of social welfare. The theoretical inter-relationships between particular ideas about welfare and particular sociological models of state and society will be drawn out where appropriate. The emphasis here will be on understanding how particular ideologies or models of state and social policy presume certain understandings of the development of and the role played by post-war welfare up to and including the present period. The chapter considers in detail the ways in which social democratic orthodoxy influenced thinking about and the provision of social welfare before moving on to consider challenges to that orthodoxy in social policy and the reasons for their emergence. This chapter is concerned with developing an analysis of social policy in the pre-Thatcher period. Consequently, we consider the supposed social democratic hegemony in post-war social policy and the major Marxist and neo-liberal critiques of that preeminent model. In Chapter 5, we move on to look at other, more recent challenges to social democratic social policy. There, we cast the intellectual spotlight on the new Conservatism and new Labourism, as well as considering the feminist critique of social democratic welfarism.

The social democratic orthodoxy: welfare and bureaucratic collectivism

The views considered here are drawn from a collection of writers whose work has emerged over some sixty or so years. Some are social science academics, some are politicians, some are social welfare practitioners – and some are all three. Despite differences in time and professional location which characterise this group of authors, and despite differences in ideological and intellectual emphasis within this body of work, certain core assumptions emerge. These shared assumptions, which dominated social policy teaching for much of the post-war period, have been identified in an earlier chapter but bear brief repetition before moving to a more particular consideration of the different emphases within the social democratic approach.

First, the following views of social policy are all grounded in an assumption that the state, its institutions and its functionaries are subordinate to the will of democratically elected governments. In other words, the social democratic or revisionist literature assumes that the state plays no independent – or countervailing – role in the processes of social policy development and definition of policy aims and purposes. The civil service and other state institutions are seen as simply administrative arms of government in the drafting and implementation of governmental policy. Second, there is a presumption that government decisions about the scope and nature of state intervention in social policy reflect, and are responses to, wider consensus on those issues – however that consensus has been created. Finally, social democratic views on welfare appear to accept that state involvement is beneficent in its intention and effect.

The social conscience thesis

This particular explanation of the development and objectives of state welfare can be found in much of the social policy literature that emerged in the first thirty post-war years. It proposes that state intervention in social welfare is best understood in terms of cumulative growth in the collective social conscience of the general population (and especially of the middle and upper classes). That collective conscience, it is argued, is reflected in organised state action in the social policy field. A societal commitment to relieve the problems of those in need called forth increasing levels of state welfare. The social policies thus created were therefore no less than the institutionalised expression of altruism or, as one author has expressed it, the 'obligation a person feels to help another in distress which derives from the recognition that they are, in some sense, members one of another' (Hall, 1952, p. 308). The social conscience thesis sees the aim of state welfare as the rectification of 'diswelfares' suffered by disadvantaged citizens. Implicit in this is a belief that state social policy can operate to create greater equality in British society.

Authors writing from this sort of vantage point included many of the most influential post-war social policy writers. Because of the immense influence of this approach, it will be considered in some detail.

Social policy development

Much of the literature which adopts this approach constructs a model of cumulative, irreversible and positive social policy development. Implicit is a belief in the primacy of rationality and morality in the ordering of social affairs. The relatively low level of state involvement in social policy until this century is explained in terms of widespread ignorance about the causes and extent of social problems. The growth of institutionalised state welfare services is understood as stemming from increasing awareness of social problems and an accompanying moral conviction that they should be resolved. The ultimate response to this collective sense of moral obligation was the creation of a welfare state by and within a benevolent, responsive and democratic state (see Sullivan, 1987; Jones, 1991, for a detailed account of pre-welfare state developments in social policy).

The enlargement of state activity into a welfare state was, from this perspective, born out of

> an era of moral shock and remorse caused by the relation of the appalling conditions of the poor shown to exist by Charles Booth's great inquiry into the *Life and Labour of the People of London* and other investigations. A sense of compassion combined with the pangs of conscience led to a middle and upper class revolt against a state of affairs that had now become intolerable. (Robson, 1976, p. 34)

The development of state welfare is seen, by social conscience theorists, as a mysterious process but one based on a concordance of ideas about the need for state intervention rather than as a process characterised by a conflict of interests between social classes and between government and state institutions. Quite simply,

> education is provided because knowledge is believed to be good and ignorance a bad thing. Disease is treated because health is looked upon as more desirable than sickness. Income is maintained because poverty is regarded as an evil . . . . (Slack, 1966, p. 40)

In other words, the development of state social policies is seen as the institutional response to a groundswell of social altruism.

Before this century, state involvement in welfare had been limited to a range of activities for the relief of poverty and disease. Such activities, as we have previously noted, were grounded in a victim-blaming analysis of social problems. These activities tended to define what we now believe to be *social* problems as the result of individual deficiencies in victims' personalities (see, for example, George, 1973, pp. 6–12, on the philosophies implicit in poverty relief programmes).

According to the social conscience writers, early-twentieth-century state social policies on income maintenance, compulsory education and health care marked a shift in the scope and nature of state intervention to resolve social problems, and were underpinned by a changed understanding of problem causation. Increased knowledge about the extent and context of poverty, and the political agitation of social reformers and the poor themselves are seen as having contributed to the social reforms of the 1906–11 Liberal governments (see Gregg, 1967, pp. 8–13, and Bruce, 1961, for a description of these reforms and the factors claimed to have influenced their enactment).

Such informed, and essentially moral, responses to the discovery of socially caused needs has, according to these writers, characterised state intervention in welfare for most of this century. The process of state provision of welfare reached its climax during the 1940s with the enactment of a package of policies which we now regard as having been the cornerstone of the British welfare state. Beveridge's social insurance scheme is argued to have been the inevitable response of opinion-formers, and ultimately of government, to a recognition that poverty was often caused by unintended interruptions of earning. The scheme provided for a basic minimum income during periods of earnings interruption and is said to have contributed to the defeat of material need (see Rodgers, 1969, vol. 2, chs 11 and 12). Further improvements to the scheme, such as the introduction of an earnings related unemployment benefit in the late 1960s are seen as responses to a consensual recognition that the transition from employment to unemployment, or from one job or skill to another, is often outside the control of the individual worker and should not consign the unemployed worker to poverty.

Similarly, the health care plans of the wartime coalition government, and Bevan's National Health Service Act (1946), can be seen as the reaction of government and state to the generally recognised need for a universal health care system which should be free at the point of need for all British people (Sullivan, 1992). Once the full extent of the health needs of the population had been established, no government could have acted otherwise, even if that meant tackling the problem of the relationship of the medical profession to the state (see, for example, Rodgers, 1969, vol. 2, p. 50 or Brown, 1976, p. 48).

The 1944 Education Act, which ensured compulsory secondary education for all, and the introduction of comprehensive secondary education in 1965 can be seen from this perspective as the institutionalisation by state and government of the principle of equality of opportunity which had taken root in the minds of the British people. The 1944 Act followed and responded to the evidence of government commissions, trade unions and teachers' organisations that existing arrangements were socially divisive and wasteful (see, for instance, Sullivan, 1992). The comprehensive reorganisation can be seen as developing from a groundswell of popular opinion that the post-1944 system was not achieving the hopes of the majority of the British public for equality of educational opportunity (see Parkinson, 1970; Rubinstein and Simon, 1973; Reynolds and Sullivan, 1987; Jones, 1991; Sullivan, 1992).

The picture that emerges is quite clear. The development of state social welfare intervention is seen as resting on and stemming from the growth of social conscience among the population in general. This collective conscience promoted a rational and moral response from government and state in enactment and implementation of social policies. The social conscience thesis is founded on a belief in a powerful, well-informed and rational state, the existence of which precludes the idea of continuing serious injustice.

The aims of social policy
For the social conscience theorists, the aims of social policy are unproblematic. For Slack (1966, p. 93), they are threefold:

(a) the prevention of suffering, premature death or social ill;
(b) the protection of the sick and vulnerable from dangers and pressures which they cannot withstand; and
(c) the promotion of the good of the individual and society.

As we might expect, this paradigm brooks no conflict between individual protection and prevention from ill, on the one hand, and the needs of society on the other. The assumption is that the needs of individuals and society are likely to be essentially similar in a society characterised by political consensus. However, even in a society which is essentially harmonious and just, problems such as poverty and disease occur. Many such problems are perceived as having roots in temporary societal malfunctions, and the aims of state welfare was to rectify these peripheral diswelfares.

Citizenship and social policy

This view of social policy is similarly rooted in social democratic approaches to the state. Like the social conscience approach it sees state intervention in welfare as developing from consensus. Unlike that approach, however, it sees consensus as being forged out of sometimes conflictual processes. Like the previous approach it sees state social welfare as operating to alleviate diswelfares. However, unlike that approach it recognises the creation of equal social rights as justifying economic inequality. The work of T. H. Marshall and C. A. R. Crosland will be considered here, although a number of writers share all or part of the perspective (see, for example, Parker (1975) for a thoroughgoing attempt to study social policy development from this perspective).

The development of social policy
In a seminal article entitled 'Citizenship and social class', the late Professor T. H. Marshall (1963) outlined a model of social policy

development which has had considerable influence. The model owes much to the nineteenth-century economist Alfred Marshall's hypothesis that there is a kind of human equality associated with the concept of full membership of a community. Full membership of a community, or society, is – according to the later Marshall – contingent on possession of three sets of citizen rights: civil rights, political rights and social rights. In contemporary society such rights may be defined in the following way (Marshall, 1963, p. 74):

civil rights are those rights concerned with individual liberty and include freedom of speech and thought, the right to own private property and the right to justice;

political rights are primarily those rights of participation in the political process of government, either as an elector or as an elected member of an assembly;

social rights cover a whole range of rights from the right to a modicum of economic security through to the right to share in the heritage and living standards of a civilised society.

State provision of social welfare was perceived by Marshall as part of the package of social rights which are one component of the citizenship rights. The development of a complete bundle of rights which is the property of all social classes is a relatively recent development. In approximate terms, the formative period for the development of each set of rights can be set in one of the three last centuries. In the eighteenth century civil rights, especially those of equality before the law, were extended to wider sections of the population than had hitherto been the case. In the nineteenth century and early twentieth century, political rights previously limited to the aristocracy, were extended first to the middle classes, then to working class men and finally to women. In the twentieth century social rights, previously available only to the destitute (and then on unfavourable conditions through the operation of the Poor Law), were extended to working people – in the form of selective social welfare provisions – and then, through the creation of a universalist welfare state to the whole population (Marshall, 1963, pp. 77–82).

Thus, this approach might be understood as presenting the development of state social welfare as a unilinear and inevitable

cf deserving & undeserving poor

process. Such an interpretation, however, does this approach less than justice. The roots of citizenship rights are traced back through history and the extension of these rights seen as extensions in the British democratic tradition. However, social rights – including state welfare provision – are seen as having emerged out of a democratic process, ultimately leading to consensus over social and political affairs but which included conflict between classes and genders.

Marshall argues that the movement for equality of political rights, including Chartism in the nineteenth century and suffragism in the early twentieth century, developed from a determination to extend the rights of all citizens beyond equality of civil rights. Similarly, the establishment of universal political rights and enfranchisement contributing, for example, to the election of working people's representatives to Parliament, aided the struggle for equality of social rights. These social rights, enshrined in welfare state policies, included the right to a modicum of economic security (through the income maintenance system), the right to share in the living standards of a civilised society (through policies of full employment and the health system) and the right to share a common cultural heritage (through the education system) (Marshall, 1963, pp. 84–6).

Although the extension of rights at each stage has been accompanied by political struggle to achieve those rights, the effect has been, at every stage, to mould a new consensus on rights reaching its climax in the extension of social rights. This having been achieved, social rights (education, health and income maintenance rights, for example) advanced the individual's ability to fully utilise their civil and political rights.

This citizenship-democracy model was given further substance by the Labour intellectual cum politician, Anthony Crosland. In a speech reproduced in a collection of essays published towards the end of his attenuated life, he located the movement for comprehensive secondary education within Marshall's citizenship model.

I believe . . . this represents a strong and irresistible pressure on British society to extend the rights of citizenship. Over the past three hundred years these rights have been extended first to personal liberty then to political democracy and later to social welfare. Now they must be further extended to educational equality. (Crosland, 1974, p. 194)

Social democratic views of the state and government are overt in Crosland's analysis. The consensus on rights has roots in a democratic tradition. It may, at times, have been forged out of struggle and conflict but once that consensus had emerged governments inevitably responded to an irresistible groundswell of opinion and the state machinery aided the expansion and implementation of social rights.

The aims of social policy

The citizenship theory emphasis on the creation of equality of rights did not, however, imply the creation of material equality through redistributive social and economic policies. On the contrary, Marshall's analysis saw equality of social status as legitimising economic inequalities. For him, it is no accident that the growth of citizen rights coincided with the growth of capitalism as an economic system. For economic rights are indispensable in a market economy. This is so because they permit individuals to engage in economic struggle for the maximisation of profit through the right to buy, own and sell. Political rights may have redressed some of the power imbalance between the social classes in capitalist society but social rights – by peripherally modifying the pattern of social inequality – had the paradoxical, but utilitarian, effect of making the social class system less vulnerable to change (Marshall, 1963). Social rights accorded community membership to all – and thus made all citizens stake-holders in capitalist society – without effecting any fundamental redistribution in income or wealth. Social welfare raised the level of the lowest (through income maintenance schemes, education, health care systems and the like), but redistribution of resources, where it occurred, was horizontal rather than vertical. In the British welfare state, inequality persisted but the possession by all citizens of a package of social rights created a society in which no *a priori* valuations were made on the basis of social class or social status. For Marshall, then, the aims of social policy and service provision include:

(a) incorporation of all as members of the societal community;
(b) modification of the most excessive and debilitating inequalities of British society; but
(c) the legitimisation of wider and more fundamental inequalities through this process of incorporation.

Similarly for Crosland, the aims and objectives of welfare state policy were not primarily those of equality through redistribution. For him, social equality, even if desirable, could not be held to be the ultimate purpose of the social services (Crosland, 1956, p. 148). Rather, the aims were to provide relief of social distress and the correction of social needs. Inequalities would, he believed, be lessened as a result, but the creation of equality was, at most, a subsidiary objective of social democratic social policy (Crosland, 1956). Indeed, in an earlier contribution to the debate on welfare, Crosland made his views on welfare state aims even more explicit:

> The object of social services is to provide a cushion of security . . . .
> Once that security has been provided further advances in the national
> income should normally go to citizens in the form of free income to
> be spent as they wish and not to be taxed away and then returned in
> the form of some free service determined by the fiat of the state.
> (Crosland, 1952, p. 63)

The creation of a welfare state in the 1940s had, in Crosland's view, substantially, if not completely, satisfied the need for universal and full membership of the societal community. The objects of state welfare provision were to cushion insecurity and to ameliorate excessive inequality rather than to promote equality. The idea of state welfare as the shock absorber of inequalities in capitalist society is one which is also found in some of the Marxist views on welfare. The difference is that, while Marshall, Crosland and others see this function as an appropriate one, it formed part of the Marxist critique.

What springs from the social democratic literature then, is a set of theoretical perspectives and a practice that served well enough for much of the post-war period. The emergence of a rational/moral consensus led to the development of state social welfare and to the creation of a welfare state. That welfare state aimed to, and to some extent succeeded in, ameliorating social diswelfares and dulling the edges of inequality. It did so by providing hitherto unprovided services and by according a form of non-material equality to citizens. It emerged from a capitalist system which, civilised or not, gave and received succour from welfare. Social democratic welfare created, in other words, a 'hyphenated society' (Marshall, 1971). Social democratic, mixed economy, welfare capitalism appeared to work well enough for thirty or so years (see

Mishra, 1990; Sullivan, 1992; and Chapter 1); but even during social democracy's fair-weather period storm clouds were gathering. Though tempestuous weather was to be postponed until the mid-to-late 1970s, social democratic ideas and practices in social and economic policy were the objects of radical challenges even during the welfare state heyday.

Radical challenges to social democracy: the capitalist state and social policy

Throughout the welfare state period, social democratic concepts of the state and social policy were disputed by the Marxist left. The Marxist critiques identified a problem which, it was alleged, social democratic theory overlooked. The issue at stake was the problem of the capitalist state. As we shall see below, Marxists, unlike their social democratic half-siblings, believed the capitalist disposition of the state had significant impact on the development and aims of social policy.

Marxist approaches to social policy in this period were explicitly linked to socialist views about the state in capitalist countries. However, as we have seen in Chapter 2, there is a debate within Marxism, as well as between Marxism and social democracy, about the exact nature of the capitalist state. We shall now see that Marxist approaches to the development and aims of social policy exhibit similar differences of emphasis.

The development of social policy

One of the fundamental Marxist criticisms of social democratic welfare politics has been that it under-emphasises two essential characteristics of capitalist society: that it is a class society and that the state is, to greater or lesser extent, the organising device of a ruling or capitalist class. As far back as Marx, himself, this was the *sine qua non* of Marxist political theory. In speculating on the ability of the capitalist state to meet the needs of citizens, Marxism's originator stresses that citizen need-satisfaction can only ever be partial in a capitalist society. For Marx, the development of total welfare which provided for the needs of people was impossible under capitalism. However, the argument in some of his writings (see Marx, 1967, vol. 1, for example) that partial welfare, which provided for the satisfaction of some of the needs of people (and working class people in particular), was possible may point up an ambiguity or duality in his thought. In other words, Marx saw that piecemeal social reforms might meet some human needs while, at the same time, his overall system determinism led him to question the extent of change possible.

The example most referred to in this respect is Marx's analysis of early protective legislation in the form of the Factory Acts (1833–67) (see Mishra (1981) for a detailed discussion of Marx's views in this respect and Marx (1967) for the original argument). Marx was in no doubt that the Factory Acts constituted a serious modification of the capitalist system: the regulation of working hours posed a restriction on the employer's ability to exploit the worker. This development is seen as resulting from the struggle between the working class and the ruling class, 'the outcome of a protracted civil war, more or less veiled' (Marx, 1967, vol. 1, p. 307). Additionally, a third grouping was involved. The landed aristocracy, perceiving a conflict of interests between themselves and the industrial bourgeoisie, became instrumental allies of the working class and paradoxically a significant part of the movement to enact reform measures.

What emerges, then, is an analysis which suggests that the capitalist state intervenes partially to satisfy citizen needs if working class pressure is significant enough and threatening enough, and/or if there are divisions of interest in the capitalist class. Here we have an analysis which exposes the duality in Marx's views of the capitalist state referred to earlier. Although the central understanding of the state, in Marx's writing, is that it is simply an instrument of the dominant class (see Marx and Engels, 1967), there is also a strand of thought which suggests that the state is, or might be, relatively autonomous from the class structure.

What then of post-war Marxist challenges to the social democratic welfare state? Mandel's approach (1968) appears to draw nourishment from the red meat of Marxist fundamentalism (or system determinism). It presents us with a very simple picture: developments in social policy should be seen as reflecting changes in the nature of capitalism. In the early stages of industrial capitalism state welfare was largely absent but, where it did exist, arose from a need to bolster an economy based on entrepreneurial capitalism. Sanitation and housing policies were developed to ensure the existence of a healthy working population housed in the proximity of industrial work-places. Very little more state intervention was necessary, certainly not in the economy, as entrepreneurial capitalism would respond, almost instinctively, to market forces.

However, as the entrepreneurial capitalism of the nineteenth century developed into the corporate capitalism of the twentieth century the state was, perforce, drawn into social and economic intervention to sustain the profitability of capitalism in its new form. The capital intensive operations of large corporations required a stability of consumption of their products: corporate capitalism responded rather more slowly to the forces of the market than had its entrepreneurial forebear. To ensure stability of consumption, the state intervened to provide systems of social insurance, social security and unemployment benefit. The worker whose earnings had been interrupted accordingly continued to consume.

Moreover, corporate capitalism's drive to increase productivity, consumption and therefore profit, led to the introduction of policies for mass health and educational services so that the productivity and productive life of the worker might be increased. This sort of approach, while lacking the sophistication of other Marxist approaches which suggest a greater degree of autonomy for the state (see Chapter 2 and below), tackles social democracy head on. The need to develop state welfare systems is seen as having little to do with the establishment of a moral/rational consensus. Rather, state welfare developed to assist the development of a new phase of capitalism. More than this, social democracy makes the mistake of believing that the welfare state altered the nature and objectives of capitalism and of the capitalist state. For this type of Marxist, social democratic commitment to the welfare state is no more than acceptance of capitalist political values.

Baran and Sweezy (1968) construct a similarly deterministic model. For them, one of the features of modern post-war capitalism was that its productive potential constantly outstripped demand for its products. The social democratic, mixed economy welfare state simply provided a context for the operation of policies which stimulated demand. State income maintenance policies might, of course, be seen to be the clearest social policy illustration of this.

Social democratic social policy intervention is thus seen as having arisen from the requirements of post-war capitalism. It marked neither the end of capitalism as some on the political right had feared (Powell, 1969), nor its transformation as some social democrats had hoped and believed (Crosland, 1952). Rather it had strengthened the power and wealth of the powerful and wealthy. A social democratic interventionist state simply distinguished and was part of a new phase of capitalist development.

There are, of course, Marxist approaches which are less reliant on this sort of crude economic determinism. The social historian Saville allows for a range of other significant formative influences on the development of social policy. He sees state welfare policies as having developed, at least in part, as a result of working class agitation for better standards of health, education, housing and economic security (Saville, 1957). He argues, however, that while working class struggle might have been the engine of social policy development, post-war welfare provision represented no more than concessions made by the British capitalist class. Furthermore, the ruling class and the state tolerated only those adjustments in state activity that contributed to economic efficiency and social stability.

Thus post-war education and health policies might be seen to have contributed to the creation of a workforce made more productive because of its possession of intellectual skills and good health. Education and personal social service policies might have contributed to social stability by establishing social institutions which socialised working people into the values and norms of capitalist society.

The American writer, O'Connor (1973, 1984), similarly sees state welfare as emerging from militant working class struggle. However, he argues that the policies which emerged out of twentieth-century class struggle had the apparently perverse effect of protecting the interests of the owners of capital. Though state social welfare was precipitated by the agitation and struggle of the poor and working class, the policy forms which emerged illustrate the predisposition of the state to act as a handmaiden to a ruling class or elite. As a consequence of this analysis, the American war on poverty of the 1960s is seen as having been precipitated by the spread of civil rights and welfare rights militancy of the period. However, the policy innovations developed were of a type which reinforced the values of a capitalist society, dependent for its continuation on social and economic inequality (O'Connor, 1973, pp. 150–75). The capitalist state, in its activities in welfare, as elsewhere, has acted as the 'class conscious directorate' of the ruling class.

In this sort of model, there is no place either for ideas of welfare development based on the establishment of a rational/moral consensus, nor for the idea of a neutral state implementing the policies emerging from that consensus. Instead, it is asserted, the development of welfare state policies emerged from class struggle. Though the working class made some advances in that struggle, the policy forms which materialised were more consistent with the interests of capital than with the concerns of labour, and were drafted and implemented by a state possessing no autonomy from the capitalist class.

Some Marxist writers, though equally critical of social democratic theory, have reacted against this bias towards system determinism. In their writing, the development and aims of welfare statism are seen as rather more complex. They are seen from within an analysis of society and state which emphasises the contradictions intrinsic to capitalist society and the possibility of some degree of relative state autonomy from the capitalist class.

Among the more significant contributions to this strand of Marxist thinking was work that appeared towards the end of the period of political consensus (for instance, Gough, 1975, 1979; Corrigan, 1979; Ginsburg, 1979; Leonard, 1979). These writers understand the post-war mixed economy welfare state as exhibiting a degree of relative autonomy from capitalism.

Gough, for example, argues that while some major twentieth-century welfare interventions have been made in pursuit of ruling class self-interest, others have represented and sprung from wider interests. At times, the threat or actuality of popular discontent and mass struggle have forced, or encouraged, the state to act in the interests of a wider constituency than the ruling class. At other times, a congruence of interest between the two major social classes has occurred and specific welfare interventions have emerged out of this convergence of interests. So the development of mass education in capitalist societies is seen as having issued from capitalism's need for an educated workforce; state provision of education can, therefore, be seen as illustrating the state's handmaiden role to capitalism at a particular historical point and in particular circumstances. The presence of popular discontent and the threat of mass struggle can be seen as precipitating such reforms as the 1911 Unemployment Insurance Act, and such state action can be viewed as demonstrating the state's capability of acting in the interests of sections of the population other than the ruling class. Health, education and income maintenance policies developed during and since the 1940s can be regarded as stemming from an identity of interest between capital and labour: capital requiring a healthy, educated and physically efficient workforce, and labour demanding access to a civilised quality and standard of life (Gough, 1975, pp. 72–6; 1979, pp. 64–74).

Similarly, Ginsburg appears to suggest that the welfare state emerged as an uneasy settlement of the usually contradictory forces of capital and labour:

> the welfare state is not . . . an untrammelled achievement of the working class in struggle . . . nor is it viewed as an institution shaped largely by the demands and requirements of the capitalist economy. The welfare state has been formed around the contradictions and conflicts of capital development. (Ginsburg, 1979, p. 2)

Pre-Thatcherite, post-war social security policies, for instance, can be regarded as having developed to aid the reproduction of a surplus labour force but also, if secondary, to mitigate poverty. In other words, post-war social policy developed out of political contradictions. In welfare, the state acted relatively, if not totally, autonomously from the interests of the dominant class.

A somewhat different argument was constructed by Offe, who sees state welfare as having developed, in some part at least, because of the heterogeneous nature of ruling classes. He understands the state as sandwiched between two inherently antagonistic influences (capital and labour). Because the state generates large amounts of income from private capital, and because the social provenance of senior state personnel is similar to that of the owners of capital, the state is usually inclined to protect the interests of the capitalist class. Much social welfare intervention (including health, education and income maintenance) should therefore be seen as having developed because the state has acted to promote those interests. According to this author, the post-war state operated in a tension between the power of capital and the strength of labour. When it was confronted on welfare (as on other issues) by mass political action (or the threat of such action), it possessed the ability to display a degree of relative autonomy from the class formation. Policies which emerged at such times arose because of – rather than despite – working class action, and were more attentive to the interests of the whole population than policies which were developed in other circumstances (Offe, 1982).

Marxist understandings of social policy development in the process of welfare development differ in the emphasis placed on the needs and interests of capital on the one hand, and the activity of the working class on the other. They differ also in their assessment of the extent to which the post-war welfare-capitalist state might be seen as autonomous of ruling class interests.

There is a resulting difference in emphasis in their views about the aims of state welfare. All are agreed that the welfare state has reproduced the social and economic relations of capitalist society. There is, however, significant disagreement about the extent to which welfare policies might also and paradoxically have provided some degree of welfare for their recipients. It is to a presentation of these different accounts that we now turn.

The aims of social policy

Welfare as the handmaiden of capitalism
For a number of authors, the aims of welfare are conceptually unproblematic. If state welfare developed out of corporate capitalism's need to provide stability of consumption and increased productivity and profit, then the aims of state welfare are clear. For Mandel, as for Baran and Sweezy, the system that created welfare also determined its objectives. Twentieth-century corporate capitalism required stability of demand for its products and, once demand has been stabilised, increased productivity of those products. Welfare met these twin demands by providing a modicum of economic security so that, even in unemployment, people continued to consume, and also by developing policies in education and health which contributed to increased productivity and to an increase in the productive life of workers. Welfare-capitalism therefore performed a servicing function for the capitalist economy.

Both Saville and O'Connor amplify this analysis. Saville sees capitalism as having two main preoccupations: economic efficiency and social stability were satisfied by post-war welfare capitalism which worked as a 'shock absorber' for capitalist society. Like Mandel and Baran and Sweezy, Saville sees state policies in the areas of education, health and income maintenance as having contributed to economic efficiency and stability in post-war Britain. Unlike them, he also perceives capitalism's need for social stability and legitimacy. Consequently welfare, by providing a measure of economic security, education, health care and the like, advanced system integration, especially in times of unrest or potential unrest. It did so, incorporating a potentially radical and rebellious working class into capitalist society, by providing albeit reluctantly, an extension of social rights. The possession of these social rights eroded working class radicalism, evoked social obligations to maintain the *status quo* and achieved the social stability and legitimacy required for the perpetuation of capitalism, (Saville, 1957, p. 11).

O'Connor also attributes twin aims to post-war welfare capitalism. For him, they were capital accumulation and legitimisation. Social democratic social policy is seen as having helped to achieve both of these aims. State welfare policies are seen primarily as legitimising mechanisms: the state involved itself in expenditure on projects and services which were likely to preserve social harmony. Social work services were provided by the state to promote conformity and value congruence in a society exemplified by value conflicts and potential class warfare. Anti-poverty programmes, such as the American 'War on Poverty' and the British Community Development Projects, were introduced as palliatives at a time of militant unrest about the plight of the urban poor. The programmes themselves implicitly saw the problems of poverty as caused by the fecklessness and flawed moral values of the poor. O'Connor therefore sees such programmes as having legitimised structural inequality in capitalist society by attempting to change the values of the poor.

State welfare, though primarily contributing to a process of legitimisation, may also, according to O'Connor, have contributed to the process of capital accumulation. Obvious examples here are education and income maintenance policies (O'Connor, 1973, pp. 169–75).

? levels g state - ? need to distinguish

Post-war state welfare intervention was intended to serve as a handmaiden to capitalist society. It serviced the economic needs or the social needs of capitalism, or both. The state in providing welfare services and developing welfare policies displayed relatively little, if any, autonomy from the ruling class or elite whose interests state social welfare served.

The contradictory nature of welfare and relative autonomy

The system determinism of the authors cited above is tempered in the writings of Gough, Ginsburg and Leonard. For them the development of the British welfare state was rooted in contradiction, and the welfare state itself manifested some degree of relative autonomy from capital. Correspondingly, the aims of the welfare state were also contradictory. The prime function of state welfare was, it is argued, to service and reproduce capitalist economic relations and capitalist values: '[the social security system] is concerned with reproducing a reserve army of labour, the patriarchal family and the disciplining of the labour force' (Ginsburg, 1979, p. 2).

However, welfare operated – albeit secondarily – to provide a modicum of security. So that while the provision of public housing policy was 'directed towards regulating the consumption of a vital commodity for the reproduction of the labour force' it was, subordinately and contingently, 'an attempt to provide secure and adequate accommodation for the working class' (Ginsburg, 1979, p. 2).

Gough argued that state welfare policies had the paradoxical role both of control and containment of the working class and of providing satisfaction of some of the needs of that class (Gough, 1979, p. 66).

What Leonard (1983) describes is a dialectic of welfare: the ability of the post-war social democratic state at one and the same time to protect capitalism and to provide some measure of welfare to its recipients is at the core of these writers' work. For them, the exact form which welfare takes and the balance of interests served by welfare is dependent, in large part, on the balance of class forces at the time of development. Welfare has functioned in more or less progressive ways dependent on the relative strength and stability of capital on the one hand, and labour on the other. The state's relative autonomy from a capitalist class has been more pronounced at times when that class, or fractions of it, are most vulnerable. Policies developed by the state at such times, like the early social insurance provisions or the post-war National Health Service, operated more obviously to provide partial welfare than did policies formed when capital was more stable. The role of welfare is always significantly constrained and directed by the relationship of the state to the owners of capital. However, the conflict between the interests of capital and those of labour are reflected in the contradictory aims and objectives of social policy.

Significant differences of emphasis exist in Marxist writing on welfare. Specifically:

1. Welfare development is seen either as a result of political struggle between social classes (real or threatened) or as stemming from the needs of capitalist society.
2. The post-war welfare state is conceptualised either as merely the 'class conscious directorate' of the ruling class, or, in other Marxist writings, as relatively autonomous from that class, though significantly constrained by its relationship with that class to act in its interests.
3. The aims and objectives of welfare are consequently seen as either to service capitalism and ensure system integration and social integration, or, on the other hand, to include sometimes contradictory goals.

Radical challenges to social democracy: social policy and the radical right

Throughout much of the post-war period, what we now recognise as radical right politics and neo-liberal economics had little effect on the development of social and economic policy. Right-wing adherents to the policies and principles associated with these politico-economic phenomena seemed like latter-day John the Baptists preparing the way for a false Messiah and a bogus millennium. All this appears to have changed, especially after the election of the first Thatcher government in 1979. Thereafter, the radical right exercised significant, though far from complete, influence on government policy formation and implementation.

Their views, associated with promotion of a market economy, have enjoyed considerable exposure in the last decade or so and contributed to a crisis of legitimacy for state-provided welfare. However, the foundations for the recent work of radical rightists – Green (1982), Minford (1984), the modern Institute of Economic Affairs (IEA) and the like – were laid in this earlier period.

Like some of the Marxists, the earlier theorists of the radical right (among them Hayek, Friedman, Peacock and Powell) constructed a powerful critique of state social policy. This critique was accompanied by explicit prescriptions for state involvement in welfare.

The development of social policy

Writers from the radical right present the development of state welfare as an unfortunate occurrence. For them, almost all state intervention in post-war social and economic affairs is to be regretted. Following Hayek (1949, 1980), the prophets of the new right have asserted that the natural state of humanity is one in which citizens are free from regulation by the state (Hayek, 1980) and unconstrained in the expression of individualism (Hayek, 1949). Such emancipation from state regulation presumes the existence of a measure of inequality in society but, for these writers, freedom and substantive equality stand in direct contradiction to each other and equality must be sacrificed in the service of freedom (see George and Wilding, 1985, pp. 21–41, and Mishra, 1984, pp. 26–64).

If state intervention in general is regarded as having interfered with the natural order, how do these writers explain its development? For Boyson, a sometime political confederate of Mrs Thatcher, the development of state welfare is to be understood within a sort of great man theory of history. The welfare state was created by well-intentioned, compassionate reformers (Boyson, 1971). Or, put another way, 'The welfare state has been fraudulently created by well meaning but misguided reformers capitalising on the aspiration of an unthinking public' (cited in George and Wilding, 1985, pp. 36–42).

In essence, most writers who adopt this approach either follow Dicey (1962, p. 259) in arguing that state welfare developed as a result of the susceptibility of public opinion to the collectivist ideology of proponents of welfare, or argue that the collectivist ideas, which justify state regulation of social and economic relations through welfare, have their source in pressure groups or trade unions rather than in individuals. In any event, they concur with Hayek about this capturing of public opinion by collectivist ideals occurs because 'Though the characteristic methods of collective socialism have few defenders left in the West, its ultimate aims have lost little of their attraction' (Hayek, 1960, p. 256). Once public opinion consolidated around the need for welfare, the state, itself a creature of collectivists, acted to institutionalise this in a systematic and ever larger network of welfare provision.

Aims of social policy

In this challenge to social democratic orthodoxy, the aims of state social policy are seen as almost entirely detrimental to the development of a free society which protects freedom of choice and promotes innovation in industry, commerce and public life. The post-war welfare state created a society in which individual responsibility for actions was vilified. The effect of this state of affairs was to encourage social disruption, resource waste, economic inefficiency and the obliteration of individual freedom. State welfare became one, though not the only, step on the 'road to serfdom' (Hayek, 1944).

For Boyson, the welfare state produced a 'broiler society' which sapped the economic and spiritual incentive of people:

> A [welfare] state which does for its citizens what they can do for themselves is an evil state: and a state which removes all choice and responsibility from its people and makes them like broiler hens will create the irresponsible society. In such an irresponsible society no one cares, no one saves, no one bothers – why should they when the state spends all its energies taking money from the energetic, successful and thrifty to give to the idle, the failures and the feckless. (Boyson, 1971, p. 9)

State welfare provision had the twin effects of removing freedom and thence responsibility, and of dampening down incentive.

The specific and pernicious objectives of state welfare were seen as:

(a) the promotion of social grievances;
(b) the wastage of resources;
(c) economic inefficiency; and
(d) the obliteration of individual freedom.

The welfare state fostered social disruption by translating needs into rights. The provision of universal services (health and education, for instance) was seen as taking no account of the extent of need for free services. Instead it provided blanket coverage for the minority of needy but also for the majority who could provide or finance services for themselves. Resources were therefore spread thinly and animosities created between potential recipients of overburdened state services (see Powell, 1972).

Free state services also led to resource wastage. Even if administered universally, state social services have limited resources. However, at nil price demand is infinite. Provision of free state services therefore stimulated demand which it could not meet. The providers were unable to evaluate which demands for service were justifiable and which were not. The consequence was the misallocation and waste of resources (Lejeune, 1970).

Resource waste was also engendered by consumer dissatisfaction with state services. Because services were administered centrally, consumers, it is argued, experienced a sense of alienation from such externalised services. This alienation was channelled into calls for increases in resources and the post-war state responded by providing more welfare to stifle 'a continual deafening chorus of complaint' (Powell, 1966, p. 20).

Although this may not have been the intention of the social democratic founding fathers, state social welfare also operated to promote inefficiency. As central state services are, in effect, a government monopoly sheltered from the price and profit mechanisms of the private market, there was, throughout the welfare state period, a tendency towards profligate and unnecessary expenditure. Monopolistic social welfare also acted as a disincentive to innovation and experimentation which might have led earlier to more efficient provision of social welfare (Hayek, 1973, vol. 1, p. 14).

Equally importantly, the post-war welfare state removed individual freedom and responsibility. The provision of state education, for instance, compelled parents to send their children to schools in particular areas and with uniform curricula. For most of the post-war epoch, parents were therefore denied the freedom to choose what sort of education provision might best meet their children's needs (see Friedman, 1962, Chitty, 1989). For the radical right state welfare provision represents back-door state tyranny and socialism by stealth. The post-war social democratic welfare state interfered with and perverted the 'natural' workings of a market economy. It stimulated demands which it could not meet and it stripped the individual of freedom and responsibility. The result of such a trenchant analysis was, of course, a set of prescriptions for welfare which suggested a significant reorientation and restructuring of state involvement in welfare.

Prescriptions for welfare

The ultimate aim for early writers within this tradition seems to have been the dismantling of the welfare state. They looked forward to a time when a market economy, generating economic growth and increased national wealth, would prevent extreme inequality of wealth and income. In such a situation, it was believed, an efficient free enterprise system could dispense with state intervention; individuals and communities could and should provide and finance private welfare.

Even short of the ultimate, these anti-collectivist writers argued for radical changes in state welfare provision. Specifically, they recommended a reduction in the scope of social services, a reduction in the level of financial state benefits, for local rather than central control of welfare and for substantial privatisation of services. In short, they aimed, in the words of George and Wilding (1985), for 'a residual, means tested, locally administered welfare state'.

The basic reasoning went like this. Policies of subsidy and rent control in housing have a number of effects. These include housing shortage caused by the reduction of price below that which current levels of supply and demand create (Lejeune, 1970, p. 32) and lack of individual freedom because rent control and housing subsidies make people subject to the decisions of others (Hayek, 1980, p. 344).

One solution recommended by anti-collectivists in the late 1970s and early 1980s was the encouragement of home ownership. This would reintroduce the ideal of individual freedom and re-establish the primacy of the market as a regulator of supply and demand (see Seldon, 1981, p. 71–86) as well as giving home-owners a stake in *status quo* capitalism. Another suggested solution was that housing subsidies, in whatever form, should be more rigorously means tested so that only the very worst off would benefit from state involvement in housing policy.

Similarly, according to this tradition, health and education services, when provided by the state, are ill conceived. Removal of price mechanisms has led to low quality service. The burden of taxation on the population, necessary to finance the services, has proved a general disincentive to work and innovation. The suppression of consumer choice in welfare state services has been a denial of consumer freedom.

Pre-1980 radical right, anti-collectivist proponents therefore suggested the removal of state-provided universal services in health and their replacement by compulsory insurance schemes (Harris, 1972, p. 76). In education, for example, it was suggested that the state should provide financing for the service to ensure universal education coverage but should ensure freedom of consumer choice through a system of parental choice of schools (Boyson, 1971, p. 8; Harris and Seldon, 1979).

The pre-Thatcherite radical right then advanced a view of welfare which dismissed a substantial role for government and which prescribed, instead, a minimalist and residual role. How then, did this sort of approach develop in principle and practice, during the 1980s and the 1990s? In principle, because radical rightists continued to prescribe social policy aims; in practice because from 1979 until the present the United Kingdom has had Conservative governments which have declared indebtedness to the political nostrums of the neo-liberals. This, along with other emerging challenges to the old social democratic welfare state, are the concerns of Chapter 5.

Understanding social policy
Radical challenges to social democracy in the 1980s and 1990s

The neo-liberal revival? Radical rightism, politics and social policy in the 1980s and 1990s

The 1980s has been seen as a decade of fundamental change in economic and social policy (Hall, 1979, 1988; Aaronovitch, 1981; Aaronovitch and Smith, 1981; Rowthorn, 1981; Mishra, 1984; Johnson, 1990; Sullivan, 1992; Hill, 1993, see also Chapter 1). The election of the 1979 Conservative government is sometimes seen as a political watershed. Of particular interest to us is that Conservative governments over fifteen years have been seen as profoundly changing the social policy map.

Despite Prime Minister Thatcher's apparent commitment to conflict politics and her sympathy for the radical right, consideration of the relationship between ideology and intention on the one hand, and the outcome of Conservative social policy during the fifteen years is a complex process. This complexity was hinted at in Chapter 1 where a hypothesis of long-term aims achieved by piecemeal means was floated. This chapter tries, among other things, to flesh out that hypothesis and further consider its validity.

Intentions and outcomes

For some, the intentions of the Conservative Government at the beginning of this period were patently clear. One writer believed that the Conservative party had accepted the radical right view of the Welfare state 'as an alien imposition financed by taxes from working class people for the benefit of scroungers' (Leonard, 1979), another that the 1979 Election represented 'a distinct vote against the welfare state' (Corrigan, 1979). For these writers, radical right intent was writ large in the policy ideas of the first Thatcher administration.

Clearly, there was serious consideration given to the rhetoric of rolling back the state from welfare. Nor was that concern without foundation. It is easy to spot the influence and intentions of the radical right in some of the policy ideas that emerged during the first two terms of government. It is also the case that some policy outcomes appeared to couple with those intentions. More than this, in the third term of government policy intentions and outcomes moved closer to each other than in the previous years. To this extent, at least, radical right thinking might be seen to have propelled governments into a wholesale repudiation of social democracy and all its works.

The objectives of Conservative social policy

So what were the objectives of Conservative social policy in the 1980s and what was the nature of the assault made on social democratic principle and practice?

Johnson has recently argued that during the 1980s the UK welfare state has been reconstructed (Johnson, 1990). He sees the aims of Conservative social policy as having been threefold:

(a) to increase privatisation;
(b) to attack the power of the local state; and
(c) to promote inequality (pp. 7–34).

In other words, there appears to have been a reasonably close relationship between radical right principle and Conservative government policy practice. The mainstays of social democracy, as theory and as practice, were eroded by a Conservative policy process inspired by, or indebted to Hayek, Friedman, Powell and the contemporary torch-bearers of radical right economic and social thought (see Harris and Seldon, 1979, 1987; Minford, 1984). In turn, the 'big ideas' of the social democratic past, a mixed economy, the responsibility of the central state to intervene, and the accountability of local government were turned on their head – or so it appeared. Social policy was used by the Conservatives in a way consistent with the free-market principles. However, implicit in Johnson's inquiry is the premise that Conservative aims were not to dismantle the welfare state, as some (Corrigan, 1979; Gough, 1979; Leonard, 1979) had thought at the time. Rather the objective was to transform it. This, of course, is a very fine distinction because the argument from the political left consisted, and to some extent consists, of the counterthesis that transformation and destruction have amounted to much the same thing. A consideration of the development of social policy during the 1980s might help us to clarify the arguments.

The development of Conservative social policy

Despite the growth among nascent Thatcherites of a radical right approach to politics in the mid-to-late 1970s, social policy prescriptions in the first Thatcher election manifesto suggested that the announcement of social democracy's death was premature. As I have argued elsewhere, the 1979 Conservative party programme cannot be regarded as a manifesto for a radical change of direction for social policy (Sullivan, 1989, 1992). The programme on which the first Thatcher government was elected contained relatively little evidence of an attempt either to transform or to destroy the welfare state (Sullivan, 1989, pp. 36–40). What concerns us here, however, is what developed after that first Conservative victory had been won.

Certainly, the policy agenda was expanded to contain new ideas. For instance, by 1982 the Central Policy Review Staff (CPRS) – central government's 'think-tank' – was suggesting radical changes in health, education and income maintenance policies including the replacement of the NHS by a private health insurance system, the end of public funding of higher education and the de-indexation of a number of social security benefits. That these particular changes, which were in line with radical right thinking and promoted by radical right political agencies, failed to materialise was in part the result of public outcry (Riddell, 1983; Taylor-Gooby, 1985) rather than a repudiation of radical right political ideas. Other changes did occur however.

Health policy

As we have seen in Chapters 1 and 2, health policy turned out to be a political minefield. On returning from the United States in 1982 after a fact-finding mission about private health insurance, the then Secretary of State for Health, Patrick Jenkin, was convinced that the British public would not tolerate wholesale private provision. Recognising the political reality that the NHS remained 'the most popular component of the welfare state' (Papadakis and Taylor-Gooby, 1987, p. 40) the Conservatives, on one reading at least took:

> a succession of Granny's footsteps tiptoeing away from the universal, publicly-funded comprehensive health service hoping that no one [would] be sufficiently alarmed by the noise to ask the questions of principle raised by each step. (Cook, 1988, p. 6)

That is to say, although the radical right intent of government social policy remained intact, gradual and piecemeal reforms of the NHS became the preferred means of achieving radical objectives.

The move to private practice

Readers with sufficiently long memories will remember that the 1974–79 Labour governments had introduced a policy of phasing out private practice from the NHS. It established a Health Services Board to direct a phased run-down of private beds. The first Thatcher government set about reversing the effects of this move with relish. The Health Services Act (1980) abolished the Board and made the Secretary of State responsible for ensuring the presence of private beds in NHS hospitals.

Though the battle was entered with relish, the victory was somewhat pyrrhic: the passage of the Act, in fact, coincided with the growth of private hospitals which took increasing numbers from the private patient 'pool'. However, the insinuation of private practice into the NHS system was achieved in other ways.

In 1980, the government introduced changes to consultants' contracts. These changes made it possible for consultants to increase their private practice without incurring disadvantageous conditions in their NHS practice. The new contracts allowed a greater proportion of a consultant's salary to be earned in private practice before forfeiting any NHS salary. They also reduced the proportion of NHS salary forfeited once the cut-off point had been reached (Higgins, 1988; Johnson, 1990, pp. 70–2). According to Higgins, the result of this change was that there was a significant increase in the number of consultants who, while working on full-time or maximum part-time contracts for the NHS, engaged in significant private practice. As Higgins notes:

> In a situation where there were so few wholly private practitioners and where the service was so firmly consultant-led the potential for the expansion of private practice was dramatically changed. Although the increase in private health insurance and the availability of new private sector facilities were important factors, their contribution to the changing scene would have been marginal were it not for the radical restructuring of consultants' contracts and consultants willingness to take on new work. (Higgins, 1988, p. 87)

Further encouragements consisted of tax breaks for employees and employers participating in employer-funded private health insurance schemes – a development which led, *inter alia*, to the introduction of private health insurance schemes run by some major trades unions! Here then was a clear breach of a social democratic politics of welfare. More than that, this first Thatcher innovation in health policy enshrined the idea of choice in welfare. Patients were to be given a wider selection of health care options. As such, this change clearly demonstrated the links between Mrs Thatcher's new Conservatives and the thinkers of the radical right.

Private insurance and private facilities

Along with the growth in private practice came the growth in private insurance schemes and private provision. By 1988 over 10 per cent of the population were covered by private health insurance, double the proportion covered in 1979. This apparently small proportion is, in fact, deceptive because health insurance schemes have tended to exclude older people and those with chronic illnesses and disabilities.

With government encouragement, three provident associations dominated the health scheme: British United Provident Association (BUPA), Western Provident Association and Private

Patients' Plan took the lion's share of the private market. Towards the end of the 1980s, however, a number of for-profit companies have entered the private health market, competition has become fierce and a market in health looks, to some, a near reality. It is, however, a very limited market. Despite the government's target of 25 per cent of the population to be covered by private insurance by 1990, the most recent figures are well below that.

This steady but unspectacular growth in private health insurance was accompanied by a growth in the provision of private facilities. Notwithstanding the changes introduced by Conservative governments in the 1980s, the number of private patients treated in NHS hospitals has declined continually over the last 20 years. This has less to do with the number of pay-beds available in the NHS, which have remained relatively constant during the 1980s, than with declining rates of occupancy of those beds. Instead, private treatment has increasingly occurred outside the NHS. Some commentators see the stimulus for this growth of private facilities as stemming from the attempt by the Callaghan government to phase pay beds out (see above). Whatever the reason, and this certainly appears to have been one influential factor, the acceleration of provision of private facilities in the 1980s was substantial: 'while in the 1970s around three out of every four private patients were treated in the NHS, the reverse is now the case' (Griffith *et al.*, 1987, p. 79).

This growth in facilities has been accomplished through the intervention of two kinds of hospital facilities: commercial hospitals and those run by not-for-profit organisations. By the late 1980s they were catering for roughly equal numbers of patients with the two major UK providers, Nuffield (a charitable trust) and BUPA growing more quickly than the others but with American for-profit corporations attempting to break into the market (see Higgins, 1988).

Notwithstanding the appearance of an incipient free market in health, the private health sector has grown as a result of its dependence on the NHS as well as its competition with it. First, the NHS acts to increase the potential profitability of private medicine. It does so because it has to treat all patients seen to be in need of hospital care. This includes the bulk of patients who would not, in any event, be able to pay for their treatment and leaves the private sector to concentrate on the more exotic or more profitable acute cases.

Second, private hospitals profited during the late 1980s from work diverted to them by district health authorities (DHAs). This has largely, though not exclusively, been the result of central government waiting list initiatives in 1987 and 1989. In both of these years the Department of Health made extra funds available to district and regional health authorities for the purpose of reducing patient waiting lists (£25 million in 1987 and £33 million in 1989). In many though not all cases, waiting list initiative monies have been used to contract out work to the private sector. This was particularly the case with relatively uncomplicated minor operations.

Third, the NHS has increasingly subsidised the private medicine business through its use of 'agency' doctors and nurses in locum capacities. The cost of locum consultants has been, on some occasions, equivalent to twice the salary of an NHS consultant (*The Guardian*, 17 June 1987).

Last, the NHS heavily subsidises the private sector through its training of medical personnel. Doctors and nurses transferring from NHS to private hospitals bear no responsibility to repay the NHS for their training, nor is there any expectation that their new employers will be involved in reimbursement.

Here then, the Conservative governments of the 1980s appear to have acted with some political adroitness. Reorganisation of the NHS allowed the growth of private provision within the context of a service still formally committed to collective provision. Additionally, of course, the very existence of collective provision was used to prop up private medicine. Social democracy was challenged here by sleight of hand.

The NHS and the internal market

Policy developments in relation to the growth of a private health sector implied, as we have seen, repercussions in the NHS prompted by innovations external to the service. Throughout the 1980s Conservative governments also introduced measures intended to make the internal workings of the NHS analogous to the workings of a private corporation.

Of most significance was the creation of an *internal market*. The internal market idea was a brain-child of the IEA and the right wing of the Conservative party, and found favour with the Premier. It was promoted in the late 1980s by an ultra-right-wing group of MPs known as the *No Turning Back Group* (which had been established to protect the radical right ideas that had informed the policy-making of government during most of the 1980s) in the following way:

> Particular hospitals and particular areas should be able to specialise, with patients being referred to whichever can provide the cheapest or best service. Excess capacity should be traded across district boundaries instead of having empty places in one location accompanied by shortage in another. (No Turning Back Group, 1988, p. 20)

This move exposes clear political and ideological preferences. First, it was and is seen as increasing *competition* in the Service with hospitals competing with each other to secure contracts for work from DHAs. Second, it was seen as improving *efficiency* in the Service. Efficient hospitals with lower unit costs would reap the reward of more contractual work from DHAs. This would have consequences not only for them, but would also act as an incentive to less efficient hospitals to improve efficiency levels and avoid the financial penalties that such a market place in health creates. Here we see the ideological assumptions of the Conservative government: competition and efficiency are inseparable bedfellows. The post-war NHS had been inefficient *because* it did not operate in a health market-place. Monopoly provision had bred waste and the introduction of both external competitors and internal competition was intended to create a service more responsive to consumers and more efficient in its activities. The resonances with the radical right in general and with Powell (1972) in particular are clear. The destruction of service monopolies was seen as imperative to choice, efficiency, effectiveness and consumer influence.

What, taken together, do these changes signify? On one reading they might be seen as fitting in with the destruction of the welfare state thesis. After all, substantial changes did occur in the Service which sometimes made it difficult to recognise as Bevan's NHS. Of course, it wasn't. The changes that have been considered were profound. We need to understand those changes not only in the context of some sort of Thatcherite political project but also appreciate that, while falling short of the plan to annihilate the NHS and replace it with a private health insurance scheme, these led to changes consistent with radical right ideas. A programme of *restructuring* appears to have replaced the proposed devastation of the NHS. That restructuring was intended to move towards achievement of the same goals as abolition.

Whatever the intentions then, it is, or seems to be, the case that the outcomes of Thatcher governments' policies on health have been to graft free-market features onto the existing form of the NHS. To what extent is it possible to apply this thesis to other welfare state services?

Education policy

The *Thatcher effect* was certainly evident in other areas of the welfare state. In education, substantial underfunding in the first two Thatcher governments (DES, 1983; Flather, 1988) were accompanied during the third term by changes at the level of organisation and curriculum. In the case of primary and secondary education, the most significant restructuring came during this later period. Legislation was introduced to allow primary and secondary schools to 'opt out' of control and funding by their local education committees (LEAs) and to take on grant maintained status with financing coming directly from the Department of Education and Science (DES) (or in Wales from the Welsh Office). Under the provisions of the Education Reform Act (1988), opted-out schools can hire and fire their own staff and determine terms and conditions of employment. In common with their LEA counterparts, they are self-managing with school governors occupying a pivotal management role. Unlike schools in LEA control they are unaffected by LEA policy decisions (Simon, 1988; Dale, 1989; Sullivan, 1991).

Significant changes have also occurred at the level of curriculum. During the third term of government, Mrs Thatcher's administration introduced a national curriculum with the overt intention of standardising and rationalising the learning process of pupils. This has proved contentious, not because of the stated aims but because of a set of alleged covert aims which include the intention to 'rid the school curriculum of subjects regarded as potentially politically or morally subversive: peace studies, political or civic education, sex education and sociology' (Sullivan, 1989, p. 67).

A further change introduced under the Education Reform Act (ERA) has been the right of parents to opt, through the parental preference scheme, for the school of their choice for their children. Here, as in health, a form of consumerism lies at the heart of the changes.

Further and higher education policy has also introduced some major changes. Expenditure on higher education has been substantially cut in the last ten years or so: government expenditure on universities being cut by 15 per cent between 1980 and 1990 (DES, 1990). As a result of these economies, 19 per cent of university posts were lost between 1979 and 1988 (Association of University Teachers, 1989) and up to twelve universities have faced bankruptcy during the period. As early as 1984 the University Grants Committee, a quasi-governmental, though formally independent, body which administered government funding to universities before its replacement in the late 1980s by the Universities Funding Council was claiming:

> these cuts are so severe that great harm has been done. Academic planning has been disrupted, morale has been impaired, thousands of young people have been denied university education, confidence in government has been shaken and will be difficult to restore.
> (University Grants Committee, 1984)

The intention behind this apparent underfunding of the university sector of higher education was clear: universities should establish closer links with commercial and industrial enterprises, should bid for research and consultancy contracts and should seek to make good the short-fall in government funding through access to this sort of private funding. This policy direction was also followed in the polytechnic sector where increases in the number of students attending these institutions had not been matched by increases in government funding. This had led to reductions in the level of spending per student of around 20 per cent between 1980 and 1984, and had prompted the National Advisory Board on Higher Education (a sort of Higher Education Funding Council for the polytechnics) to warn as early as 1984 that '[it is] not possible to achieve the triple objective of access, maintenance of standards and a continued downward move of the unit of resource' (National Advisory Board for Higher Education, 1984).

By the third term of Thatcher government, these financial strictures had been supplemented by wider policy considerations. So the Education Reform Act (1988) removed from university teachers' contracts the clauses which had hitherto granted them permanent job security. This has been seen by some as an instrument to effect not only the ability of universities to keep within restricted budgets by making academics unemployed, but also as a means of controlling, through the fear of termination of contract, the freedom of expression of politically dissident academics. The issue here is not whether such a development was to be applauded or regretted. Rather the issue is that, as with the most recent NHS reforms, the Thatcher government was prepared to arbitrarily change the terms and conditions of professional workers in order to increase accountability.

In the education sector, as in the NHS, Conservative social policy has sought to elevate the position of the consumer, to restrict, where necessary the power of the professionals, to marginalise areas of learning seen as inappropriate or subversive, and to introduce, through the opting-out mechanism a market-place in school provision. This last intervention is ideologically very interesting because it appears, on one analysis at least to epitomise radical right thinking about social policy.

First, the reform introduces the notion of consumer choice. Parents as consumers, both as represented on school governing bodies and as the final arbiters through ballot, are the key actors, at least in theory, in choosing whether their school applies for grant maintained status. Second, the reform can be seen as being at the cutting edge of a radical right inspired campaign against large welfare bureaucracies – in this case LEAs. This is so because opted-out schools free themselves from the policy direction of the local council and in so doing break down the power of those welfare bureaucracies. Third, opting out can be seen as consistent with a long-held desire of the radical right to privatise welfare because many regard the opting-out provisions as a half-way house not only to the recreation of selective education but also to private education. This is so because it is believed that grant maintained schools will, in the short-to-medium term be allowed to become independent schools.

Yet, here – that is, in education provision – as well as in relation to health policy, if the policy intentions were indebted to the influence of the radical right, the outcomes have been less than entirely consistent.

Despite a distaste for the comprehensive organisation of secondary education and legislation (Education Act 1980) freeing local

authorities from the compulsion to provide non-selective schooling, the Conservative governments of the 1980s have failed to
mount a full and direct attack on the comprehensive principle. On
empirical grounds this might be intelligible. Much of the evidence
suggests that the very inequality of opportunity, that right-wing
Conservatives believe to be a natural corollary of naturally different abilities, has been as much an outcome of the comprehensive system as it was of the bipartite system (Ford, 1969; Reynolds
and Sullivan, 1987). On an ideological level, the governments' caution is more surprising.

Comprehensive secondary education, whatever the empirical outcomes, represents one of the ideological totems of social democracy
and the politics of consensus. Crosland's promotion of the policy
idea, Boyle's tolerance of the development of the comprehensive
school and Labour's stewardship of the reform are all partly explic-
able if we remember that one of the assumptions underlying consensus politics was that the achievement of equality of opportunity
through social policy was politically uncontentious. The Conservative right, on the other hand, believed the idea that equality of opportunity could be achieved to be fatally flawed and to have resulted in
educational opportunities having been offered to more pupils than
could possibly make use of them (Boyson, 1971; Harris and Seldon,
1979). Ideologically, then, the failure of Thatcher governments to
act more forthrightly is apparently less intelligible.

Similarly, although in 1990 the third Thatcher government, almost in its death throes, planned the introduction of more overt
competition between universities and institutes of higher education by privatisation of the institutes and by suggesting the removal
of the binary divide between them, the DES remains heavily involved in the funding of both sectors. True, both groups are competing in an educational quasi-market-place to increase student
numbers in line with the government ambition to see 25 per cent of
the age population entering higher education by the turn of the
century. True, government funding is now disproportionately dis-
tributed so that institutions which more adequately meet
government-inspired performance criteria are rewarded and those
which do so less adequately are penalised. True also, that pressures
undoubtedly exist to sell wares in the so-called real world.

These are all changes associated with the Conservative governments of the 1980s. That these changes are detrimental to higher

education is yet to be demonstrated, if indeed it can be. That they constitute fundamental perversion of the purposes of education as a social service must also remain open to question.

Taken in the round, changes in education policy amount to a restructuring or reorientation of education: local authority stewardship of the school system has been weakened; parents, if not pupils, have emerged as important actors in the implementation of policy plans; and the status of professionals has been diminished. In this respect, Conservative governments of the 1980s kept faith with radical right nostrums on social policy.

Yet where are the other policies promoted by Mrs Thatcher's confederates on the Conservative right in the 1970s? The idea of education vouchers to promote consumer or surrogate consumer choice has been dusted down several times in the 1980s only to be placed back on the shelf. The idea of abolition of the maintenance grant scheme, a scheme introduced in 1963 as a result of the Robbins principle, had a similarly unhappy passage on to and then off the policy agenda. The idea was that such a proposal would limit entry to higher education to serious students only, that is those who were prepared to pay for the privilege. It would encourage a sense of personal responsibility for progress and thus underline the inappropriateness of the nanny state. In the event, of course, one unsuccessful attempt to introduce this reform, resisted by parents and government backbenchers, was followed by a much lesser strain, holding grants at their 1990 level and introducing partial individual responsibility through the means of top-up loans.

Education was restructured. However, the idea that education, especially higher education, is an individual responsibility rather than a citizen right has yet to be promoted successfully. Indeed, governments of the 1980s have seemed to withdraw from it. In this area of social policy, then, we might want to argue that once more prominent radical right ideas have been bolted on to a previous social democratic social policy agenda.

Other social policy areas

A similar story can be told for the other social policy areas. In income maintenance, for example, the idea of the radical right, of the IEA, of the Centre for Policy Studies (CPS) and of some gov-

ernment ministers including the Premier, was that state social security provision should be removed and replaced by a compulsory
private insurance scheme. That idea was never implemented. Instead, we have seen the abolition of some benefits (Sullivan, 1989, p.
43), the de-indexation of others (Sullivan, 1989, p. 44), and a keen-
ness to bring social security fraudsters to justice (Sullivan, 1989, pp.
45–6) in the early part of the 1980s. In the last half of the 1980s we
have seen, following a Social Security Review, the revision of the
social security system. This has taken the form of making some
erstwhile mandatory social assistance benefits discretionary and reducing the value of many social insurance benefits (Johnson, 1990
and Chapter 1). The clear intent, and to some extent outcome, of
these changes has been to reintroduce a principle of reduced eligibility for the administration of benefits to what Murray (1990) sees as
a growing British underclass. That outcome is significant in policy
and in wider political terms because it questions the eligibility of
certain sections of the population to full citizen rights. It is still some
way, however, from abolition of the state system although it needs
to be said that the correlation between policy intent and outcome
appears to be closer here than in the cases of health and education.

The Personal Social Services area has also seen change. It has,
tduring the 1980s, become the victim of the twin processes of
underfunding and increased responsibilities (House of Commons
Select Committee on Health and Social Services, 1984, cited in
Sullivan, 1989, pp. 77–9). They have also seen a change in role and
orientation. Following the then Secretary of State's warning in
1984 that local authority social services departments should make
better use of the voluntary social welfare sector and should take on
a strategic enabling role rather than attempt to provide all necessary services themselves, plans were developed which eventuated
in the community care proposals of the National Health Service
and Community Care Act (1990). These proposals, implemented
in 1993, signal not only a shift away from institutional care in
health and social services, and the creation of a supposed seamless
web of care in the community. They also establish in the social
services field, the same sort of purchaser/provider split as has been
introduced in the NHS. Local authority social services departments will continue to identify, fund and plan statutory services.
Those services will be provided by a variety of agencies of which
local government departments will be but one.

Here again, the changes were far from insignificant. Competition was to be introduced into the provision of community care as it had been into the provision of institutional care in the 1980s. Then private residential homes had burgeoned. Now community care was to be provided by a consortium of care agencies including the NHS, local government and the voluntary sector. Resources would remain limited because, in line with Conservative right-wing thinking, families and communities were to bear a greater portion of front-line care. Though significant, the reforms, past and present, have done little to diminish the demand for social workers – 'revolutionaries on the rates', Boyson called them in a newspaper article. The response to Brewer and Lait's provocative question, *Can Social Work Survive?* (1981), appears to be in the affirmative but only by adopting the role of care management rather than case work.

With the possible exception of income maintenance policies, it is often said that only in housing was the full extent of policy intentions matched by outcome. In their 1979 Election manifesto (Conservative Party, 1979), the Conservatives had pledged that, were they returned to power they would legislate to make it mandatory for local authorities to offer their tenants the opportunity to buy the houses they presently occupied as rentees. This pledge was kept to the letter and tracts of local authority housing stock became part of the private market. This was part of what Mrs Thatcher liked to refer to as people's capitalism and such has been the political success of this piece of housing policy, whatever its social costs, that by 1987 it had become a bipartisan political commitment (Labour Party, 1987).

However, in some other respects, the correlation between expressed political values and political action in housing was less close. Interestingly, despite the ideological component in the policy of council house sales, the Conservative governments of the 1980s seemed less than bold in the application of free-market principles to general housing policy. So, despite high demand for housing in the south-east of England in the mid-1980s, supply lagged far behind because of apparent government unwillingness to overcome constraints.

It is also the case that, regardless of support and encouragement from the right, Thatcher governments also failed to introduce free-market principles into the issue of private rents. The CPRS had proposed in 1982 that the government should take action to de-control rents and allow the market to settle what constituted an economic rent for a property. Despite Mrs Thatcher's later advice to an increasingly dissident Chancellor of the Exchequer that 'you can't buck the market', the CPRS proposal, though studied, was rejected.

It is true, of course, that in Thatcher's last term the government introduced legislation, the Housing Act (1988), which allowed for groups of council tenants to transfer their properties to the owner-ship and management of private management companies. This provision introduced the possibility of further erosion of the public rented sector and, as the Act allows for the possibility of tenants themselves forming housing management cooperatives, it permits a solution which appears consistent with Conservative emphases on both property ownership and self-help. None the less, taken as a whole, housing policy under three Conservative governments in the 1980s appears to point in no consistent political direction. On the one hand, radical right political commitments appear to be present in the policy of council house sales and the associated drastic fall in local authority housing starts – 130,000 in 1976, 40,000 in 1983 (Taylor-Gooby, 1985). However, neither the de-mands of a right-wing ideology nor the extent of housing need appear to have been dominant factors in the framing of a general housing policy.

Some conclusions

In May 1979 the Conservative party formed a new government. During the 1980s they were to win two further elections by sub-stantial margins. The 1979 government headed by Margaret Thatcher, as were the other administrations until she fell to a palace coup in late 1990, found consensus politics anathema – or so, at least, it seemed. The political project announced loudly and proudly at the dawn of the Thatcher experiment was to reassert the place of conviction politics, to rehabilitate neo-liberal eco-nomic principles and social conservatism. In relation to the welfare state this was seen as requiring the removal of the state from large tracts of welfare provision, replacing it with provision admin-istered by the individual, the family or the community, or by a variety of private and charitable agencies acting on behalf of citizens and sometimes funded directly by them. As we have seen, the vision in this form was not to be translated into reality.

Despite the chronic political weakness of Labour, the major opposition party for most of this period, the welfare state was neither destroyed nor replaced. This is not to say that fundamental changes were not introduced. Shifts in the direction of welfare occurred during the 1980s in each of the areas we have reviewed above. The NHS has become less of a monopoly provider of services than it had been hitherto. It has been the subject of policies intended to make it function like an effective business: the introduction of internal markets, of external competition and of a degree of privatisation. In education, the private, or quasi-private, sector has been strengthened. Consumers, or more accurately surrogate consumers – parents, have been empowered to make choices about the status of their local schools and about where they wish their children to attend school. These choices had previously been the province of professional educators or administrators. Additionally, the higher education sector has been visited by policies intended to make it more efficient, more accountable and more responsive to the needs of society, or at least to commerce and industry. Similar policy patterns have emerged in other social policy areas.

It is quite clear that in both intent and outcome the politics of welfare have been transformed or restructured. Policies have been imposed as a result of conviction rather than consensual agreement. Those politics have become more partisan and have signified the rejection by leading Conservatives of a politics of consensus in welfare. This is, none the less quite a different proposition than the claim that the intentions and outcomes of Conservative social policies have been consistent with each other. As we have seen, they have not.

So, how do we set about explaining the apparent disjuncture between the extensive aims of Conservative social policy at the beginning of the period and the ostensibly more limited policy outcomes?

It is at least possible to argue that the political gap between intention and outcome is less wide than appears to be the case. Though it is true, on one reading, that the early rhetoric sits uncomfortably with the outcomes of Conservative social policy, this is far from the whole story. What seems to have happened, in my opinion at least, is the modification of aims. Instead of presiding over the wholesale destruction of state welfare, Conservative governments have incrementally changed the nature of the welfare state (also see Chapter 1). In crude terms, that change can be described as the introduction or attempted introduction of the market into social welfare or, as it has been described in Chapter 1, managed competition. That change documented above has had a number of political and practical ramifications.

From client to consumer

The first of these has been the development, by the new Conservatives, of consumerism in welfare. In other words, there has been a not entirely unsuccessful project to change the relationship between welfare services and the users of those services. It is widely acknowledged that the relationship between post-war welfare services and their users was one characterised by clientism. In other words, public welfare monopolies, freed from the effects of competition to provide services, retained definitional, planning and management functions within themselves. Users came to be seen as recipients of services planned for them. This phenomenon, whether in the personal social services (see Handler, 1973), the NHS (see Klein, 1983) or in any of the other services, was, of course nourished by a social democratic political tradition that emphasised the importance of experts in the planning and running of welfare services (see, Sullivan, 1991, 1994, ch. 11). Penetration of the market into welfare services aimed to change the nature of that relationship between purchasers and providers of service on the one hand, and recipients on the other.

The introduction of a patients' charter in the NHS, together with the 1990 Act and, in Wales, *Strategic Intent and Direction* (SID), call for a redefinition of the relationship between the welfare state and the patient. In this new relationship, the patient becomes a consumer and can be guaranteed not only information about treatment but also the right to contribute to the planning of user-centred services. The extent to which these strategies are currently successful is not our concern here. What is of concern is the clear political preference to introduce into the NHS the consumer/

provider relationship of market organisations. Whatever else has yet to be achieved, this move appears to have contributed to a diminution of the power of professionals to determine the shape of local health policy. It has also contributed to a move by DHAs to see themselves as patients' advocates and to act accordingly (Paton, 1991; Ham, 1992).

Similar moves are, as we have already seen, afoot in other services. While consumerism in housing (the sale of council houses and the provision for management agencies in the 1988 Act) is well established, consumerist strategies are being introduced in personal social services agencies and are at the heart of changes in all sectors of education. As with the Labour opposition (see below), the Conservatives appear to have redefined the notion of citizenship. Whereas Marshall saw citizenship as residing in the gradual increase of social rights, the Conservative emphasis on consumerism stresses, instead, individual rights. In this cession of citizenship, the *individual patient's* rights are posed against the professional power of medicine, the individual parent's rights against the wish of the education system to hold on to information, and so on. Citizenship becomes, then, stripped of its social or collective meaning.

From social welfare to internal markets

The new Conservatism has attempted to recreate welfare state clients of the social democratic epoch as welfare consumers of the 1990s. Another significant development, as we have already noted in Chapter 1 and above, is the introduction of internal markets, or the splitting of welfare bureaucracies into commissioner and provider arms. This clear departure from the social democratic past is intended to make welfare organisations more efficient and more responsive to user needs. As we have already seen, the NHS, the personal social services and areas of education are now the sites of internal markets. By separating the commissioning of welfare from its provision, Conservative governments hope to increase the efficiency and effectiveness of service. The theory here is that welfare provision will be spread more widely than in the post-war welfare state and that a range of service providers will be able to offer service for purchase from commissioning agencies (DHAs, local

authority social services departments and the like). Commissioners, acting as 'champions of the people' (Welsh Health Planning Forum, 1991), will then purchase the most effective and
efficient service irrespective of whether the provider is a state
service or a private organisation. More than this, these commissioning agencies will be able to monitor and influence service re-
sponsiveness through their contracts with service providers.

So, even though new Conservative governments have stopped
short of wholesale privatisation of welfare state services, they have
– in theory at least, and maybe in practice – broken the state
monopoly of welfare. In doing so, the idea, and maybe the reality,
of the welfare consumer has been used as a Trojan horse.

In short, the new Conservatism has transformed the nature of the
social democratic welfare state by introducing market mechanism
into social policy concerns. It has not destroyed the structure of
welfare. Nor has it yet successfully attacked the universal provision
of many areas of the welfare state (although the so-called *welfare
state review* carried out by the Treasury during 1993 might change
that). It has, however, managed to replace the practice of clientism
with the idea of consumerism and welfare monopolies with internal
markets. Though Conservative governments have clearly failed in
any project to roll back the state from welfare, they have changed
the nature of the social democratic welfare state and have moved
towards minimalist statism – although, of course, they have yet to
arrive. They may, however, have satisfied Seldon's first stage in the
privatisation of welfare. We must wait and see.

The new Labourism: the 'citizen' returns

The successful influence exerted by the new right on Conservative
governments since 1979 and the achievement of those governments in transforming the social democratic settlement, has also
led to some new (or recycled) thinking from social democrats. This
is particularly the case with the Labour Party.

Labour's thinking on social policy has moved, over the last decade, from old-style social democracy to a less than grudging acceptance of some of the changes introduced by Conservative
governments. During this process a sort of citizenship theory has
re-emerged.

If we look at Labour's social policy agenda in the late 1980s and early 1990s, the following trains of thought emerge. First, there are certainly elements of the old social democratic approach in its strategy for social policy. In its strategy document on health (Labour Party, 1991), it side-swipes at the Conservatives' emphasis on efficiency strategies in the NHS. It declares that 'most of what appears as inefficiency [in the NHS] is the product of underfunding' (1991, p. 2). Second, and notwithstanding this standard response, even here there is substantial recognition of the durability and acceptability of some elements of the Conservatives' health service reforms. Of most significance, perhaps, is Labour's intention, despite earlier ambivalence, to retain the split between the commissioner and provider in the NHS and personal social services, a crucial element in the emerging welfare pluralism. This is clearly an acknowledgement of the potential success of this mechanism in improving service. Its clear acceptance of the commissioner/provider strategy as a mechanism to improve effectiveness and efficiency suggests, though it does not ensure, that managed competition, perhaps in a more restricted form, is as attractive to the policy elite in the Labour party as it is to the present government. This, alongside another acknowledgement of Conservative social policy, might suggest that Labour, like the Conservatives, sees a degree of competition in welfare as likely to assist not only its commitment to peg direct taxation at its present level but also a commitment to meet need.

For several years, Labour has accepted the retention of the general management system introduced into the NHS in 1983, following the report of Sir Roy Griffiths (1983). Taken with the commissioner/provider split, Labour sees the system as achieving a goal that has eluded health ministers since Bevan, the subjugation of professional interest to patient need. Put crudely, Labour, like the Conservatives, expects managers and DHAs to determine health need and to provide services to meet that need. The role of doctors and other medical professions will be to apply their technical expertise to that task in a political climate that decreasingly accepts them as health planners as well as technicians.

Labour's move towards Conservative social policy aims is clear in other social policy areas as well. As we have seen, a commissioner/provider split in personal social services, planned under the provisions of the National Health Service and

Community Care Act, has become common political property as has the elevation of the role of the voluntary organisations in both planning and providing care (Labour Party, 1990).

Large differences in approach to social policy remain between the major parties of course. The 'new' Labour party continues, for now at least, to reject opt-out schemes in education and health and to wish to draw a clear demarcation line between services regarded as public and those regarded as private. It is pledged to work to force the reversal of underfunding in the heartland services of the welfare state: health, education and social security.

It had, none the less, moved a great distance even before the watershed election of 1992. Its policy aspirations in the early 1990s appear to take account of the shifts in public opinion documented in recent commentaries on welfare provision. Labour may, in crude terms, have become more aware in the late 1980s of the complexities contained within public attitudes to welfare. Those complexities embrace not only the strong support for heartland welfare state services, which – or so I have argued elsewhere (Sullivan, 1992) – have acted as a brake on Conservative social policy plans, but also ambivalence to social security provision and some universal benefits (see also Papadakis and Taylor-Gooby, 1987).

So how should we present the new Labourist approach?

Taking health and personal social services as their focus, a body of opinion within the party has suggested that welfare pluralism plus the commissioner/provider split amounts to an improvement in citizens' social rights (Marshall, 1963). The argument goes something like this. There is a clear need for the retention of purchasing activities within the structure of a welfare state (DHAs and local authority social services departments). This is so because a public body responsible for assuring the health and welfare of the population, but shorn of the responsibility to provide all services, has many advantages. The major advantages are:

1. Such bodies will be able to concentrate on issues of preventive care as well as restorative care as a result of their distance from provision activities which, when structurally indivisible from purchasing activities, lead to conflict of interest.
2. The distance of purchasers from providers will assist the former to take a critical look at existing provision.

3. The purchaser is thus liberated to choose whatever provision works rather than retaining an interest in supporting those who have traditionally provided services.

It is, of course, this last argument that suggests support for, or tolerance of, private provision existing alongside and being used by welfare state services.

What appears to be emerging is a fusion between Beveridgian welfare state concepts and ideas about a so-called 'opportunity state'(Sullivan, 1990). Both in a Fabian Society lecture in 1985 and in a speech on the eve of the 1987 general election, Kinnock, then leader of the Labour party, tried to construct a defence for restructured Beveridgian social democracy in new political times. His argument was that a major function of the 'old' welfare state was that it had increased opportunity. In his 1987 speech he illustrated his point by a question addressed to his audience at the Welsh Labour Party Conference. 'Why', he asked, 'am I the first Kinnock to get to university and why is Glenys [Kinnock] the first woman from her family to have done the same?' The answer was the welfare state and its widening of access to higher education. The speech was significant because it presented the welfare state as the 'opportunity state'. The argument being constructed was that it had only been possible to meet *individual aspirations* through *collective provision*. This appeal to the opportunity state is interesting because, while appearing to mine the rich seam of conventional post-war British social democracy and particularly the Crosland legacy, it also represents an acknowledgement of the changes wrought in United Kingdom social politics by the Thatcher experiment. In other words, there is an attempt to present, under the cloak of the old social democracy, a move from the old emphasis on the collectivity to a new emphasis on the individual. The welfare state is to be nurtured because it aids individual development. Taxation for collective provision is simply the investment to be paid for individual protection and progress. This formulation, and its development since 1987, heralds of course the return of the citizen to Labour social policy. Equality, fraternity and liberty are about the individual. They constitute the social and political rights accorded to citizens, *as individuals*, in a civilised society. Collective politics are simply the most effective and most moral means of providing individual rights. A revamped citizenship theory, *pace*

Marshall, or perhaps more accurately, Crosland, has been the bridge used by the Labour Party to cross from old-style social democracy to a partial acceptance of changes in welfare wrought by Conservative governments.

This move has been reflected in many of Labour's policy documents in the late 1980s. During this period, the party has carried out a policy review as part of the process of rehabilitating the party in the eyes of the electorate after a period in the early 1980s when it had appeared to be controlled by its left wing. Those documents that concentrate on welfare issues (Labour Party, 1989, 1990, 1991) are noteworthy because they stress the concern of the party with individual issues such as liberty, freedom of choice and consumerism that had been colonised through much of the 1980s by right-wing Conservatism in government.

The task addressed in these documents has been economically expressed by Labour's former deputy leader, Roy Hattersley. In a short essay written at the end of the 1980s he argues that the responsibility of a future Labour government will be to 'provide and popularise an acceptable theory of distribution that is both consistent with egalitarian principles of socialism and with a modern economy' (Hattersley, 1989). Decoded, this amounts to an acceptance not only of much of the change wrought in methods of economic management in the 1980s, but also of some of the directions in social policy followed during this decade. It is also, of course, a re-working of Marshall in new conditions. The aim of the new social democracy is to create a sort of equality that is consistent both with its political past and with the retention and development of market capitalism. It is this project that has spawned Labour's *Social Justice Commission* and it is a concern with equality of accord rather than material equality that appears to be the engine driving Labour social policy development in the early 1990s.

In important respects, then, old-style social democracy is dead. New Conservatism influenced, though not fully determined, by the radical right, has – in welfare as elsewhere – transformed the debate about and the practice of welfare provision. In doing so, it has not only created a new sort of Conservatism, but also forced Labour into a new Labourist position. That position is one in which citizenship has been used as a conceptual bridge from Fabian social democracy to a sort of market socialism.

CHAPTER 6

Changing social services
A study of the demise of old-style social democracy

In the last two chapters we have traced the apparent rise and fall of social democratic social policy and its partial replacement by a new Conservative approach. That approach has been influenced by a twentieth-century revisitation of classic liberalism and has wrought significant changes in the welfare state. This chapter considers, in greater detail, the changes that have occurred in one area of provision.

Here we look at policy changes in the personal social services since World War II and attempt to make connections between those changes and deeper ideological and empirical changes in state theory and state activity.

Prelude: social work before the welfare state

Before getting into the meat of the chapter, it is useful to consider the roots of post-war state intervention in personal social services (PSS). This is so because some recent critics of Conservative social policy have characterised it as heralding a return to the social and political values that nourished pre-war non-interventionism in welfare.

Most welfare historians trace the origins of modern PSS back to the middle of the nineteenth century. Some appear to see a positive and unilinear progression from the tradition of Victorian philanthropy through to co-ordinated state provision in the twentieth century (Woodroofe, 1971). The ideology of the Poor Law (itself of much earlier origin) which marked the provision of help in the nineteenth century – dividing the poor into deserving, and therefore worthy of philanthropic action and undeserving to be punished for their feckless behaviour – is seen by some as also permeating the attitudes and activities of twentieth-century state welfare agencies (George, 1973).

Others have argued that twentieth-century PSS grew out of the failure of philanthropy. Philanthropic action, often administered by the same people who administered the Poor Law, had failed to eradicate social needs, and this failure was seen in the late nineteenth century as a blow to national prestige (Seed, 1973, p. 9).

Some recent commentators have seen the growth of private charity organisations like the Charity Organisation Society in a different light. Parry and Parry identify the evangelical Christian revival of the mid-nineteenth century as the seed bed from which social work grew and flourished (Parry *et al.*, 1979). Evangelical Christianity, with its emphasis on personal salvation, is seen as having led to philanthropic work with an emphasis on rescuing the immoral or preventing immorality. The first sign of modern personal social services appeared during the 1850s with the introduction of paid welfare workers associated with the Church and directed mainly at the moral welfare of women and girls (Walton, 1975, p. 41).

Others see the origins of state PSS as rooted in quite a different morality. For Steadman Jones (1971) the ancestry of nineteenth-century philanthropic and social welfare action are better seen in the need for a well-socialised proletariat in order to integrate all sections of the population into the structure, culture, norms and values of capitalist society and prevent social revolution. He reminds his readers of the philanthropist Samuel Smith's caution that

> I am deeply convinced that the time is approaching when this seething mass of human misery will shake the social fabric, unless we grapple more earnestly with it than we have done . . . . The proletariat may strangle us unless we teach it the same virtues which have elevated the other classes of society. (Smith, cited in Steadman Jones, 1971, p. 291)

No doubt the ideologies of nationalism, evangelical Christianity, capitalist self-interest and secular philanthropy overlapped and interacted in the early development of PSS.

Out of this hotchpotch of nineteenth-century social welfare activity developed, in the twentieth century, a series of systems of social welfare which were to exist until the late 1940s. PSS activities which focused particularly, though not exclusively, on the poor were undertaken by a strong charity sector and a variety of central and local government departments (Woodroofe, 1971, pp. 193–8). Coverage of need was patchy and the activities of different agencies were largely un-coordinated. It was not until the late 1940s that the state started to develop comprehensive social welfare services as part of a wider welfare state package.

The inception of state social work

Following the Second World War, three state PSS agencies were created. These agencies, located at the level of the local state, replaced in large part the multiplicity of independent and government agencies which had previously carried out personal social service functions. These agencies, which existed until the early 1970s and were primarily concerned with services to children, the physically and mentally sick and disabled and the elderly, carried out a range of mostly statutory responsibilities. These were especially concerned with the provision of residential or substitute care for clients in situations where home-based care was regarded as inappropriate, inadequate or damaging (see Sainsbury, 1977, for a fuller description of the services).

The reorganisation of state social work

In the early 1970s, following the report of the Seebohm Committee in 1968 and the passing of the Local Authority Social Services Act in 1970, PSS was reorganised into unified local authority departments charged with the provision of statutory and non-statutory services to those in need. Further developments in PSS have occurred through the 1980s and early 1990s. In the early 1980s, the Barclay Report (1982), recommended the introduction of *community social work* strategies. Local authority social services departments and other PSS agencies were encouraged to develop alternative practices to meet social need. Community social work presumed a movement away from the one-to-one focus of traditional social work towards the encouragement and facilitation of self-help by individuals, social networks and communities. Barclay also recommended that the social work role, for many post-war years that of therapist, should be transformed. An important element of that transformation would be a move to the role of enabler. Social workers would support and enable informal carers rather than provide all care themselves (Hadley and Cooper, 1984; Hadley *et al.*, 1984, 1987).

The most recent organisational change in PSS has followed the enactment of the National Health Service and Community Care Act (1990). From 1993, local authority social services departments have become the co-ordinating agency for community care. This has significant ramifications. First, these departments will be key players in the assessment of social need, as long-stay hospitals and institutions are closed, to be replaced by care in the community. This immense change has come at a time when form has been given to the social services departments as strategic enablers. In this new world, local authority departments have become the assessors of need and the purchasers of services rather than the monopoly providers of PSS.

The objective of this chapter is to understand these changes in modern social policy.

Personal social services in the post-war period

How then do we explain the development and objectives of PSS in the post-war, pre-Thatcher period?

It appears clear that, for two post-war decades at least, PSS policy was driven by a social democratic engine. That dynamic was based on essentially Fabian notions of human nature, professional action and the appropriate role of the state.

So some social democratic writers see services as having grown out of a developing collective conscience in modern British society. In other words, thinking about policy and its enactment were coloured by a belief in the perfectibility of humankind. Sometimes such views are made explicit.

Slack, commenting on the introduction of state social work with children, says of the Curtis Report, '[it] was based on a *new and more sympathetic* approach to human need. Emphasis was laid on the differences of each child and his value as an individual' (1966, p. 111, my emphasis).

Post-war PSS reflected, in large part, a commitment to meet need through the activities of government and state: 'whenever or wherever a social service is introduced it is to meet a need that has, whether soon or late, been recognised as real or unmet' (Slack, 1966, p. 93).

Or, as Titmuss suggests: 'As the accepted area of social obligation widened, as injustice became less tolerable, new services were separately organised around individual need' (Titmuss, 1963, p. 21).

The development of services for children and young people illustrates the social democratic social policy project well. A common theme in the literature is that social legislation in the period we are considering, developed out of 'a widening and deepening knowledge of need' (Barker, 1979, p. 178) and was part of a continuous and cumulative process evolving 'constantly . . . in the direction of greater generosity and wider range' (Barker, 1979, p. 178).

So the Children and Young Persons Act (1963), which sanctioned preventive social work to combat the need to receive troubled or troublesome children into local authority care, and the 1969 Act of the same name, which laid down a framework intended to minimise the number of child and young adult offenders appearing before courts – and saw a treatment or welfare model as more appropriate than a justice model in such cases – are both seen as prime examples of social democratic social policy. They appeared, at least at the time, as manifestations of the informed reactions of a benevolent state.

Social workers and others had become increasingly convinced, in the post-war years, that the causes of many problems associated with childhood were of a social or familial nature rather than located within some sort of individual pathology. Consequently, it was argued that problems of children's relationships with their parents or siblings were best dealt with within the family setting. Similarly, problems of juvenile criminality, associated with causative factors wider than the individual, were more justifiably dealt with by welfare intervention than by punishment.

Such legislation might therefore reasonably be seen as humane responses, by the state, to greater knowledge about the causes of social difficulties. Evidence had been produced of a wider network of factors associated with such problems than had previously been accepted. That evidence had prompted a number of further investigations by the state and by political parties (Home Office, 1965, 1968; Longford, 1966) and had culminated in rational and moral responses in the form of social legislation to cater for a minority of people experiencing difficulties.

The reorganisation of local authority social services in the early 1970s also owes its shape to social democratic ideas. In the 20 years following the inception of a state-controlled social service system, knowledge of two kinds was amassed by practitioners and administrators in the services. First, it became accepted that the tripartite organisation of state services led to duplication of tasks and uneven coverage of need (Seebohm, 1968). Second, as we have already noted, 'knowledge' was being generated that the causes of need for a minority of the population were wider and more complicated than had previously been thought (Townsend and Abel-Smith, 1965; Longford, 1966). As a consequence, practitioners academics and sympathetic Labour politicians called for a unified service which would understand and meet the needs of the individual in relation to family, community and society (Marshall, 1975, pp. 143–64). These calls, supplemented by the reports of various government committees, and particularly the Seebohm Report, led to the reorganisation of state social work.

Post-war PSS development was in some senses at least, the result of collective commitment to meet the needs of disadvantaged individuals or groups. That commitment was itself, in large part, the result of increases in knowledge and understanding. Or so it seemed to social democrats.

What, then, were the objectives of PSS for social democrats in the post-war period?

For supporters of social democracy, PSS had limited but important objectives. Only a minority of disadvantaged people, it was believed, still fell outside the advantages conferred by a transformed and welfare-oriented post-capitalist society. Certainly, by the 1950s the aims of PSS were conceived as the 'relief of residual distress' (Crosland, 1956, pp. 85–94). Though primary poverty was believed to have been eradicated by the welfare state, residual secondary poverty continued to exist alongside the problems of physical and mental illness and disability present in any society.

The primary function of PSS was therefore to be the amelioration of such conditions.

Some 1950s commentators make this more explicit. Penelope Hall, arguing that all major social problems had been successfully tackled by welfare state policies, proposed that the personal social services should tackle more sophisticated problems.

> The most urgent problems . . . today are such symptoms of a sick society as the increasing number of marriage breakdowns, the spread of juvenile delinquency and the sense of frustration of the worker in spite of improved pay and conditions . . . that is, problems of maladjustment rather than material need. (Hall, 1952, p. 8)

If this conviction that primary need had been outlawed was shattered by the 'rediscovery of poverty' in the 1960s (Townsend and Abel-Smith, 1965), the basic approach to policy remained substantially unchanged. The aims of PSS came to include helping government more fully to understand how pockets of deprivation and need remained in a post-war society characterised by rising living standards and relative affluence (Jenkins, 1972; Joseph, 1972). Poverty and need along with a catalogue of other problems were increasingly regarded as being outside the control of the individual. However, following Crosland's view that capitalism had been transformed, problems of deprivation and need were assumed as having roots in institutions intermediate to the individual and society. Thus the aims of Seebohm departments were to include the articulation and treatment of individual problems in the context of family and community (Seebohm, 1968). These aims were also to be met by state-sponsored community development projects (in the early 1970s) seemingly established to research and then change communities and thus ameliorate or eradicate need among marginal populations (Loney, 1983).

PSS policy in the post-war period was clearly part of the social democratisation of the state and its direction was supported by both major political parties. It assumed the existence of a moral/rational consensus on need and need satisfaction. More than this, it was based on a particular view of the perfectibility of humankind and the superiority of welfare over punishment. Though dominant throughout this period, this approach had its detractors, as did the wider approach to social policy in general. Those detractors, from the left and right, mounted a searing attack on the aims of PSS in this period.

The left critique

As we would expect, during this period the Marxist left suggested that PSS policy under social democratic stewardship acted not to increase welfare but as a handmaiden to capitalism. Thus the capitalist state always safeguards the interests and development of capitalism. The post-war British welfare state therefore functioned to promote capital accumulation (O'Connor, 1973), economic efficiency and social stability (Saville, 1957), and ideological conformity (Barratt-Brown, 1972).

The place of PSS in this scheme is that of a state institution operating primarily, though not exclusively, to promote social stability and the conformity of working class people to ruling class ideology. During the period under consideration, this function had been carried out in a number of ways including the use of social case work techniques 'a pseudo-science – that blames individual inadequacies for poverty and so mystifies and diverts attention from the real causes' (Case Con Collective, 1970). Capitalism was also protected by other, seemingly more progressive, forms of social work activity such as group work and community work. These activities served simply to pathologise the group or the community rather than the individual. Social work whether practised in the form of case work, group work or community work, acted socially to integrate, or socially to control, working class people. In Corrigan's words, 'throughout the western world, states are characterised by one of the two major symbols of control in capitalist society; the tank or the community worker' (1975, p. 25). Social case work, one of the major tools in the armoury of post-war PSS, was a coercive activity which defined socially caused problems as family or individual crises (see Wilson, in Cowley *et al.*, 1977). Community work and group work are seen as ' . . . means by which society induces individuals and groups to modify their behaviour in the direction of certain cultural norms' (Gulbenkian Foundation, 1968, p. 84).

However, some Marxist writing, though critical of social democracy as theory and practice, suggests that the picture is a little more grey. During the post-war period the state was seen to exhibit limited autonomy from the British ruling class. For many writers from this perspective (Corrigan and Leonard, 1978; Bolger *et al.*, 1981; Jones, 1983), PSS in post-war Britain operated within a dialectic of welfare (Leonard, 1983).

To some, social democratic theory is at least half right: post-war capitalism was qualitatively different to its inter-war forebear. Co-ordinated services were established and operated for most of the period in a changed political atmosphere and structure. The spirit of 1945 (Jones, 1983) was sustained throughout much of the period. PSS legislation and social work practice during that period reflected the clear influence of the social democratisation of state structures and social values. State policies and social work practices, while stopping far short of the provision of total welfare, demonstrated a tendency for state provision to progressively meet some of the social needs of ordinary people as well as being concerned with containment and control (Gough, 1979; Leonard, 1983).

From this perspective, co-ordinated state services managed at one and the same time to effect the contradictory aims of meeting some of the social needs of its clients while meeting the economic and political 'needs' of a dominant class in capitalist society. Welfare state social work moved from punishment to rehabilitation. Post-war social democratic politics had provided 'the ideological climate for [the] more liberal and humane welfare theories and practices to be extended to the unorganised and impoverished dependent poor' (Jones, 1983, p. 39). However, for these Marxists at least, such changes in practice and aims represented little more than a replacement of biological determinist theories of social problem causation with a set of family pathology explanations. None the less such a shift, though limited and still ideologically useful to powerful social interests, is seen as having effected a move towards understanding social problems within a wider context than hitherto.

Policies and practices related to youthful delinquency and family problems were seen as reflecting the social democratisation of welfare. The Children and Young Persons' Act (1969) was therefore conceptualised as part of a process which tended both to liberate and control.

Here, the argument is that the 1969 Act and the reorganisation of personal social services, with which it was associated temporally and philosophically, point up both the progressive and conservative nature of PSS under social democracy. The Act and the reorganisation are seen as products of the contradictions inherent in the capitalist system. Both sought to establish the primacy of a welfare model in the theory and practice of social welfare: the Act by elevating the welfare needs of young offenders above abstract considerations of justice in sentencing, the reorganisation by promoting the idea that the new social service departments would provide for the welfare needs of all in a non-stigmatising way. At the same time both social policy developments were rooted in an ideology of family pathology which saw residual problems in social democratic Britain as the result of malfunctioning family units. Such an ideology reinforced a new form of control in social work. Individuals, previously held responsible for their own difficulties were, in late-twentieth-century British social democracy, to be subject to social control through treatment rather than punishment. They were to be controlled through the identification and policing of families – often seen as the root of problems of deviance and poverty (see Donzelot, 1980).

For all Marxists, the crucial weakness in social democratic welfare theory and practice was this. In one form or another, citizens were regarded as responsible for socially induced problems. Social democracy theorised, and social democratic welfare practice operated an ideology of pathology. If the individual was liberated from responsibility for social problems, then the family or the community took the individual's place (Clarke, 1980). If social democratic PSS policy had virtue then it was, for Marxists, in the practical implications of the move from an ideology of punishment to an ideology of treatment.

Feminist assaults

Post-war PSS policy was not simply the target of the Marxist left. Increasingly, social work services were intellectually and politically assailed by the women's movement.

Feminist commentators on the development of co-ordinated state social work services make a particular contribution to the understanding of PSS development. Put simply, these commentators underline the importance of women in the development of social work from its nineteenth-century roots through to the dawning of the welfare state. The conditions associated with the early development of social work – philanthropic concern, fear of social revolution, dented national pride, etc. – led to the provision of voluntary services staffed largely by women. That social work activity was the activity of an elite is undisputed (Brook and Davis, 1985), but for much of the pre-welfare state period that elite was female. Middle and upper class women, often unmarried but sometimes the wives of the rich, were recruited into the ranks of a social work preoccupied with the rescue of widows, orphans, prostitutes and the poor in general. As a result a paradoxical situation often arose in which, according to Wilson,

> middle class women with no direct experience of marriage and motherhood themselves took on the social task of teaching marriage and motherhood to working class women who were widely believed to be ignorant and lacking when it came to their domestic tasks. (Wilson, 1977, p. 46)

This notwithstanding, social work in the late nineteenth and early twentieth centuries became largely the province of middle and upper class women (a process well documented by Timms, 1967 and Walton, 1975). Feminist writers (including Wilson, 1977; Brook and Davis, 1985) have also been instrumental in excavating from a largely male-oriented history, the reminder that, although such social work activity was predominantly the province of women, the management committees of the voluntary organisations which administered the activity were predominantly men. In this task they have been ably assisted by some male commentators (notably, Walton, 1975).

Feminist analysis of social democracy's aims for PSS draws attention to the relationship between the state and the family in capitalist (and other 'advanced') societies. For Gieve, the welfare state in general and PSS activities in particular 'highlights the link between the state and the family and the way in which the state systematically bolsters the dependent-woman family' (Gieve, 1974). For Loney and collaborators, 'the welfare system as it stands (or totters) is utterly dependent upon a specific construction of gender' (Loney, *et al.*, 1984).

For most feminist writers, post-war welfare state social work, and particularly its family interventionist activities, reinforced women's unequal and oppressed position in capitalist society as well as reinforcing other dominant ideas. Pascall (1983), echoing many other feminist writers, sees the modern family as a deeply ambiguous social formation. Although the family may be seen as an arena where the values of caring and sharing are upheld, it is also the arena where women's dependency is nurtured. It therefore constitutes the focal point for exploitative relationships between men and women. According to many feminist writers, the theory and practice of post-war social work entrenched, reinforced and reproduced women's dependency and exploitation in the family, and perpetuated fundamental inequalities between the sexes.

To appreciate the key concepts in a feminist understanding of the aims of post-war social work, it is useful to reconstruct here the important steps in feminist arguments about welfare. One of the most influential of contemporary feminist writers on welfare has argued that the welfare state constituted 'a set of ideas about the family and about women as the linch-pin of the family' (Wilson, 1977, p. 9). As such, it was also a mechanism by which women's traditional roles as wife and mother were controlled (Wilson, 1977, p. 40). Post-war social work performed functions which both protected the interests of a dominant social class and oppressed or exploited women. It did so by constructing an ideal type of family and by monitoring or policing families which failed to conform to this ideal type.

In contemporary capitalist society such family formations also imply the creation and sustenance of economic dependency for most women. Social work, it is argued, operated as one of many state institutions which played an important ideological role in perpetuating women's dependency and exploitation.

How then did social work carry out these functions? Feminist writers may point to a large number of developments in state social work to support a view that the aims of social work were deeply discriminatory or oppressive to women. Below we outline but a few examples from the theory and practice of social work:

1. It has been argued, for instance, that the report of the Curtis Committee on Child Care (though chaired by a woman and having women as half its membership) reinforced an increasingly popular view, shared by Bowlby (1953), that the care of children was best carried out in families with non-working, dependent mothers (Brook and Davis, 1985, p. 15).

2. It is further argued that the dependant–breadwinner form of family organisation was reinforced by the subcommittee of the women's group on Public Welfare in 1948, which argued 'Fre-

quently a family can survive in spite of a weak or vicious father but it is rare that it can survive with an incapable mother' (Women's Group, 1948, quoted in Brook and Davis, 1985).

3. Social work, it is argued, has imbibed an ideology of maternal care (see Ehrenreich and English, 1979) which, in practice, has restricted women's capacity to act with approval in any role other than that of dependent wife and mother. To this end social work's concern in the 1950s and 1960s with latch-key children placed working class women especially in an imposs- ible double-bind. If such women did not work their families were often driven into poverty. If they did, they ran the risk of being labelled by social work agencies as neglectful mothers (Brook and Davis, 1985, p. 16). Competent parenting, it is con- tended from this perspective, is interpreted in social work theory and practice as competent mothering. Competent mothering implies the absence of paid work outside the home and thus economic dependency on a man, preferably in a state sanctioned dependant–breadwinner family.

4. Similarly, it is argued, problems of delinquency and maladjust- ment are often, implicitly or explicitly, conceptualised in social work as problems of malfunctioning families and often as prob- lems arising from absent, working, mothers (Comer, 1971), or as a result of child-rearing occurring outside the safe confines of the dependant–breadwinner nuclear family. Specifically, it is argued by some feminists, social work constructs a model of successful child development which implies the necessity of a 'normal' family context. Moreover, the creation of such a con- text is seen as depending on the competence (and perhaps full- time presence) of the mother (McIntosh, in McLennan, *et al.*, 1984, pp. 228–9).

5. Finally, it is argued, state policies encouraging while underfin- ancing community care of the old or sick, and social work prac- tices rooted in the concept of partnership with carers, further reinforce traditional family patterns and, in consequence, women's oppression/exploitation as carers (see Finch and Groves, 1983; McIntosh, 1984; Brook and Davis, 1985).

What emerges from this rather thematic reconstruction of feminist arguments about social work, is a view that the aims and functions of post-war social work included the crucial aims of:

(a) reinforcing through theory and practice, an ideology of the family rooted in a dependant–breadwinner form of family structure;
(b) policing families (see Donzelot, 1980; Meyer, 1983), especially those who fail to conform to such patterns;
(c) entrenching, reinforcing and reproducing the discrimination, exploitation and oppression of women in contemporary society.

A rather more complex set of issues is implied by the recent work of the feminist social scientist, Fiona Williams (1991). She draws attention not only to the ways in which social policies have systematically reinforced the exploitation or oppression of women but to the interrelationship between the major forms of structural oppression. As a consequence, PSS policy, viewed from Williams' perspective, acts most potently to reinforce the tendency of the patriarchal capitalist western state to discriminate against women who are black, working class or both. This sort of study, while pointing up the impact of social policies on women as a category, allows more sophisticated analyses of the differential effect of social policies on different groups of women.

The attack from the right

As we have seen in Chapter 3, radical right formulations see social welfare as having developed as the result of the creation of a bogus consensus on the need for state provision. Many, if not all, of the arguments adduced by proponents of anti-collectivism in relation to welfare in general were adduced in the specific cases of social work provision and PSS policy.

For the ultra-right, state provision of PSS, like other state social services, led post-war Britain towards state coercion (Hayek, 1944, p. 52; Friedman, 1962, p. 13). PSS, by according citizen rights to all sections of the population, contributed to social discord (Friedman, 1962, ch. 10) and, because of its increasing call on the public purse, to reducing economic growth and prosperity. State social work was seen as having diminished individual responsibility because it 'reduces the breadwinner's individual responsibility for his family's well being, and for the pursuit of independence it substitutes permanent mutual dependence as the much more fragile basis of mutual respect' (Bremner, 1968, pp. 52–3).

PSS provision, by superseding 'the voluntary co-operation of individuals' (Friedman, 1962, p. 13), also reduced freedom: it reduced democracy, choice, respect, the role of the family and contributed to social disorganisation.

The new right apologists of the post-war years not only attacked PSS social democratic style. In its place, they prescribed a much reduced role for state social work in contemporary British society. Instead of offering a more or less universal service, social welfare services were best undertaken in the main by the family and the community. Thatcher, echoing Friedman, argued that 'if we are to sustain, let alone extend, the level and standard of care in the community, we must first try to put responsibility back where it belongs, with the family and with the people themselves' (Thatcher, 1977, p. 83). Pre-Thatcherite apologists, then, assigned both reduction in PSS functions and changes in the pattern of PSS provision.

Personal social services and the new Conservatism

As we have seen above, the election of Conservative governments throughout the 1980s and into the 1990s has effected changes to PSS policy. Hints of this, if they were necessary, came early in Mrs Thatcher's first administration. Often citing the work of the radical right, ministers, or the Premier herself, signalled a restructuring of PSS that would involve voluntarism and residualising the state.

Such a pre-eminent role for voluntary, family or community services, and a consequential residual role for state social work is clear in the advice of Patrick Jenkin, then Secretary of State for Social Services, that

> The Social Services departments should seek to meet directly only those needs which others cannot or will not meet . . . . Their task is to act as a safety net . . . for people for whom there is no other, not a first port of call. (*The Guardian*, 21 January, 1981)

Thatcher herself told the 1981 Annual Conference of the Women's Voluntary Service that the main burden of social welfare provision should fall on the voluntary sector of welfare, with statutory social services functioning simply as residual gap fillers, underpinning the work of the voluntary sector.

The scene was set for the transformation of statutory PSS

agencies into enabling organisations. Those organisations would enableinformal carers or the neighbourhood (the Barclay Report), or act as commissioners of service in a situation where much provision was offered by voluntary or private welfare bodies.

At one level at least, the new Conservatism of the 1980s and 1990s has encouraged a return to pre-welfare state approaches in PSS. While carers get on with caring and the independent and private sectors carry out state-financed philanthropy, the state is being slowly removed from centre stage in the provision of PSS. In so doing, of course, an attempt to bury the trails of social democratic welfare, perhaps ultimately doomed to success, is being made. This marginalisation of state PSS activity also marginalises the totems of social democracy itself.

First, the idea that the state has a responsibility to meet all welfare needs has been superseded by the idea that the state's responsibility is to enable informal carers, or kin, or the community to care. Second, the professionalisation of welfare, seen by Thatcher's new Conservatives and the radical right as largely responsible for the growth of welfare monopolies, is being swept aside by the elevation of informal and untrained care. Last, the social democratic idea that individual needs are best met by collective state provision is severely dented.

Another dent to social democratic PSS policy directions can be discerned in current government statements on law and order (see *The Guardian*, 21 October 1993). The clear re-emergence of a hard line on law and order – criminals should be punished not rehabilitated, prisons are punitive institutions not resocialisation centres – has carried with it attacks on social work. A criminal justice system predicated, as it has been for the last decade, on diversion from custody is, in large part, the creation of the social work lobby. That system is to be restructured, and social work and probation activities within the criminal justice system are to be made more consistent with a punitive justice model.

At the time of writing, we appear to stand on the cusp of removal of the state from large-scale *provision* of PSS. Whether services will be further rationalised must remain, for now, a matter of conjecture. The journey so far has taken us some considerable distance from the social democratic starting-point of this and other welfare state services. We move, in the final chapter of this book, to an attempt to understand the foundation of these and other changes.

PART 3

Conclusion

CHAPTER 7

Understanding modern social policy

In the earlier chapters of this book the reader has been guided through the development of modern social policy. Specific efforts have been made to demonstrate how, for a relatively long period of time, social democratic ideas and practices of state intervention achieved almost complete dominance. In the last chapter, our attention was further focused as we narrowed our consideration to the post-war development of personal social services policy. We have also described the challenges to social democracy during both the earlier and later post-war periods and have seen how social democracy's influence has been eclipsed in the last two decades. Ultimately, social democracy appears, in part at least, to have been replaced by a form of right-wing theory and practice that has guided the making of social and economic policy over the last fifteen years. That successful challenge has replaced not only the social democracy of the Labour Party but also the revisionist Toryism of Churchill, Macmillan and Heath. Here, we move on to analyse the weaknesses in social democracy that made it finally vulnerable and ultimately too weak to see off the challenge. We then look at how its demise has led to the creation of a form of social politics which is, as we have seen in previous chapters, re-drawing the welfare map.

State, welfare and social democratic views

Readers will remember that social democratic perspectives on state and social policy are based on four core assumptions:

(a) about the nature of society;
(b) about the relationship of the state to government on the one hand and society on the other;

(c) about the social forces associated with large scale intervention-
    ism including welfare development; and
(d) about the functions of social policy.

In the wake of social democracy's eclipse, the question that
concerns us is a straightforward one. How adequate an account of
the nature of society, state and welfare, and of the development of
state interventionism in civil society does this perspective provide
and what are its crucial weaknesses?

The perspective's strengths

The social democratic perspective certainly appears to have had
two particular strengths. In the first place, unlike the radical right
viewpoint, it has an explicit theory of the relationship between the
various social institutions which make up contemporary social
structure. That is to say, it rooted its hypotheses about state,
society and social policy in a clear interpretation of political structure. Another undoubted strength is that its claims and interpretations were clearly located in discussions of concrete social
phenomena (Crosland's discussion of the dispersal of ownership of
the means of control, in Crosland (1952) or Marshall's discussion
of the historical development of citizen rights, in Marshall (1963))
rather than being carried out at the level of abstract theory. Its
strengths as an explanatory perspective of modern society, have
been outweighed by a multiplicity of weaknesses at both the theoretical and operational levels.

The perspective's weaknesses

First, it appears to have over-interpreted the scope of social consensus over social values and social actions even at the inception
of the period of mixed economy and social welfare. So, for example, Marshall (1963, p. 110) appears clearly to imply that the
introduction of compulsory tripartite secondary education in the
1940s reflected a consensus on the goal of providing a complete
package of social rights to all citizens. Other authors (Rubinstein
and Simon, 1973; Fenwick, 1976; Reynolds and Sullivan, 1987;
Sullivan, 1992) clearly delineate the degree of dissension over the

question and the form of compulsory secondary education at this time.

Second, even if we accept social democracy's theory of liberal democracy, its claim that major government policies are likely to reflect social consensus over social values and social actions is at least suspect. It is, of course, true that examples of policy-making can be found which would appear to support this contention. The reorganisation of secondary schooling in the 1960s – a major piece of educational policy-making – certainly reflected the aspirations of a wide cross-section of the British population (Benn and Simon, 1972; Rubinstein and Simon 1973; Fenwick, 1976; Reynolds and Sullivan, 1987). It is also true that examples of policy-making can be found throughout the post-war period which demonstrate that government policy is as likely to run counter to public opinion as to reflect dominant trends in it. The decision by government in the late 1940s to proceed with development of the A-bomb appears, at least on the surface, to have flown in the face of a general public sympathetic to Britain's wartime ally, the Soviet Union. Policies, in the 1980s and 1990s, of restructuring state intervention and cutting the welfare state appear to run counter to public opinion when it has been sampled (see Taylor-Gooby, 1985; Jowell *et al.*, 1989, 1990, 1991).

Perhaps the weakest element of social democratic theory, however, is the presentation of the state as the handmaiden of government. The state, it is argued, is a set of politically impartial social institutions. Government determines policy: state institutions merely execute policy. This naive political principle acted as a taken-for-granted assumption by social democratic Labour and Conservative governments in the earlier post-war period. A brief glimpse at some examples of the relationship between state and government may suffice to make us profoundly suspicious of such a proposition.

The circumstances surrounding the establishment of the Department of Economic Affairs as a new government department in 1964 provides one such example. It was clear from the 1964 election manifesto (Labour Party, 1964) that, should the Labour Party, under Harold Wilson, form the government, it was intended to establish a new economic ministry to oversee and facilitate the reorganisation of British industry (see pp. 11–12). That new ministry, the Department of Economic Affairs, would operate alongside and take over some of the responsibilities hitherto carried out by the Treasury. It is well documented (see, for example, Crossman, 1975; Crosland, 1982) that the Treasury civil service acted, at least initially, to thwart the work of the new department irrespective of the new government's wishes. If we are to believe the political diarists of the time, the established senior civil service resisted change by means which included the withholding of information from ministers. Examples of similar attempts to withhold information from government ministers, thereby curtailing policy options, and of attempts to impose the policy of the departmental civil service on ministers are documented by Crossman (1975, pp. 168–9) in relation to his tenure as Minister of Housing (1964–6). Other means by which the civil service directly influenced policy-making included the development of a civil service policy line presented with unanimity at cabinet committee meetings (Crossman, 1975, p. 198).

There are also examples, culled from the literature, of the civil service arm of the state acting consciously and in direct contravention of government policy. During the economic crisis of 1976 which led the British government to seek loan facilities from the IMF, Cabinet had decided at one point to refuse the conditions of the loan despite contrary advice from the Chancellor of the Exchequer. Notwithstanding this, Treasury officials are reported to have been negotiating the terms of a conditional loan within hours (Crosland, 1982, p. 378).

Finally, an earlier example of policy-making and of the relationship between state and government throws further doubt on the validity of the social democratic proposition. This example, relating to the reorganisation of secondary schooling in the mid-1960s, quite clearly suggests that the civil service at times acts as a direct rather than an indirect policy-making body. In 1965 the Department of Education issued a circular (Circular 10/65) to local authorities requesting them to submit plans for the reorganisation of their secondary school systems into comprehensive systems (see Benn and Simon, 1972; Rubinstein and Simon, 1973; Fenwick, 1976). It is now widely acknowledged that both the form of policy-making (circular rather than legislation) and the permissive nature of the circular (encouragement to reorganise rather than compulsion, the acceptance of a wide variety of comprehensive patterns of education, etc.) were the result of its drafting by civil service officials rather than politicians. In this case, the influence of the civil service may, indeed, be seen to have been significant in that it contributed in no small way to the failure to develop in Britain a uniform system of comprehensive education to meet educational and social needs (Reynolds and Sullivan, 1986).

The proposition that the state occupies a handmaiden role to government is, then, thrown into some doubt by a consideration of the relationship in recent times between government and civil service.

Another theoretical problem with the social democratic perspective on state and social policy is that it considerably under-theorises the place of class or social group conflict/pressure in the development of state welfare services. It is true that Marshall (1963) draws attention to the role of conflict in forging a new consensus in British society over civil, political and social rights. It is equally true that Crosland (1952) perceives the growth of the labour movement as one of the factors associated with the trans-formation of capitalism. What we might later regard as a crucial weakness in the perspective, however, is its failure to theorise the relationship between opposing social forces as dynamic rather than static. Such dialectical changes may at times lead to apparent re-treats from state welfare, at other times to increased involvement – a phenomenon which reformism has difficulty in explaining.

Further weaknesses are uncovered when we scrutinise the social democratic literature on state intervention in general and the wel-fare state in particular. The idea that state intervention in welfare was intervention of a residual nature which would underwrite equality of opportunity in post-capitalist society (Crosland, 1952, 1956; Hall, 1952; Marshall, 1963; Slack, 1966, Harris, 1987) was, as we have seen, based on a number of claims. Key among them was the claim that British society had been transformed during the twentieth century from a capitalist to a post-capitalist society. Ownership had been dispersed, the power of labour had become a countervailing force to the power of capital. Equality of oppor-tunity, partial until the mid-twentieth century, had become a near reality through the development of a welfare state.

Empirical and other studies over the last thirty years have at-tacked the foundations of this social democratic edifice. Studies of poverty and inequality in the 1960s (Townsend and Abel-Smith, 1965) demonstrated the persistence of a substantial incidence of primary poverty in British society and, despite its relative lack of penetration into Tory or Labour ideology, dented the image of poverty as the experience of an inadequate minority.

Additionally, the pattern of ownership in British society and the social values of political elites appear to have remained unchanged in the post-war period (Blackburn, 1972). The increase in labour power which was undoubtedly a feature of the early post-war period has without doubt been severely curtailed by legislation and the state management of industrial relations and industrial disputes in the last ten years. Equality of access and opportunity, one of the pillars of social democratic theories of state welfare, has been shown to be a mirage. Inequality in educational opportunity has been demonstrated to have persisted throughout the post-war period (Halsey, *et al.*, 1980). Equality of access to health care appears to have been a persistent myth (Hart, 1975; Townsend and Davidson, 1982; Doyal, 1983). Equality of access to the personal social services has similarly failed to materialise. Indeed, evidence abounds which suggests that the welfare state, inasmuch as it has redistributed resources and life chances, has done so horizontally rather than vertically and has often benefited the rich rather than the poor (LeGrand, 1982; George and Wilding, 1984).

One final and significant theoretical weakness in the social democratic perspective on state and welfare remains. It presents us with considerable difficulties in theorising the present state of welfare – be it crisis or not. If the state provision of welfare has developed, in part, as a result of the growth in collective conscience, how do we conceptualise the restructuring of the welfare state and cuts in social expenditure which have occurred consistently over at least the last decade? If society was truly transformed in the mid twentieth century, how have apparently defunct social and political values reappeared to guide the actions of state and government? One way out of this theoretical impasse may be to posit the existence of a further and retrogressive transformation in ideas about the state and state activities. Such a proposition, however, poses further difficulties with and for the classic social democratic position. While it may be consistent to argue, within a perspective which upholds ideas as one of the most potent social influences on action, that changes in state welfare provision may reflect a new social consensus, much of the social democratic literature on welfare is demonstrated to be intellectually flawed by such a theoretical sleight of hand. We may be able to explain the reversal of key elements of social welfare provision (e.g. the 1966 earnings related unemployment benefit, removed in 1982; the removal of fundamental benefits from the State Earnings Related Pension System; the continuing process of partial closure of access to higher education) in terms of an adapted social democratic position. Such an apparent retreat from welfare is, however, totally inexplicable in classic social democratic approaches.

Social democratic writers on welfare have constructed a model of state social welfare which is rooted in social democratic political philosophy and suggests that social policies are inherently benevolent as well as irreversible (Slack, 1966, p. 40; Robson, 1976, p. 34). To sustain such a model requires of us a refusal to evaluate not only the evidence of history but also the contemporary experience of state activities in welfare.

The post-war social democratic approach was, then, seriously flawed. Its actions were informed by understandings of the nature of state and society that were ultimately unsustainable. Key policy strategies aimed at equalising opportunity and access capsized, in large part because social democrats of the Labour and consensus-Tory varieties failed to understand the autonomy of the state not only from ruling elites but also from government. A failure which, as we shall see, was to be rectified by Mrs Thatcher. These weaknesses were recognised long before her accession by both the political left and right. Though their conclusions differed, as one would expect, their starting points had some similarity. Both the radical right and the Marxist left saw social democracy and the social democratic welfare state as rooted in the politics of contradiction and denial.

Social democracy: the challenge from the left

In earlier chapters readers have been familiarised with Marxist views on state, politics and social policy. Like social democrats, those writing from a Marxist perspective anchored their analysis of the welfare state in core assumptions about the nature of society and state. However, the Marxist left, far from seeing the welfare state as an equality machine, saw state social policy as protecting either the short-term or long-term interests of powerful groups within capitalist society.

The strengths of the model

As an explanatory model, post-war Marxism had considerable strengths. First, its understandings of state and society were rooted in an historical as well as contemporary analysis. Unlike social democracy, it sought to place social phenomena by establishing their place in historical patterns of social development. The dynamic of history replaces the largely static social democratic accounts in an attempt to provide holistic explanations. In consequence, post-war Marxism was able to explain Marshall's development of citizen rights in capitalist society (Marshall, 1963) in a wider context. The struggle for civil, political and social rights is understood as a struggle between social classes in which subordinate social classes sought to promote and increase their interests and influence in capitalist society. The responses of state and society to such struggles are understood as responses which ultimately protect the interests of a ruling class. The package of citizen rights which emerged over three centuries of British history constituted not only the ransom paid by a ruling class in return for social stability but also, paradoxically, reinforced the interests of those in control. The granting of citizen rights is seen, from this perspective, as contributing to the social integration of society by attributing equality of membership of the societal community to all citizens while, at the same time, legitimating wider and more significant inequalities in economic power, resources and influence.

Marxist interpretations also offer an explanation of the failure of the post-war state to achieve the aims of its founding parents. The impact of many post-war social policies has been, at best, to redistribute resources and life chances horizontally (within social classes) and, at worst, to protect and increase the allocation of resources and life chances to already privileged sections of the population (Halsey *et al.* 1980; Townsend and Davidson, 1982; George and Wilding, 1984).

If the state provision of welfare is seen, in essence, as a strategy employed to protect and reinforce capitalism at a particular state of its development, then it is not surprising that the outcomes of social policy are largely consistent with intentions.

The Marxist critique of social democracy as action and theory also provides a plausible account of the restructuring of state activities in the late 1970s and early 1980s. Capitalism had entered a new stage, in part precipitated by the increasingly difficult task of maintaining the dual processes of capital accumulation and social legitimation through state interventionist strategies (O'Connor, 1973). The development of capitalism in the late twentieth century has also included the diminishing need for labour intensive manufacturing industries. As a consequence, welfare interventionism has been removed, reduced or reoriented. Emphasis on, for example, industrial training rather than on liberal education is likely to provide the technologically proficient personnel of a much shrunken labour market. Removal of the 1966 Earnings Related Unemployment Benefit and the proposals included in the White Paper on Social Security (HMSO, 1986), and later enacted, are likely to encourage the unemployed into low paid service sector jobs. Increased social expenditure on coercive state agencies is to be seen as late capitalism's response to the potential of social unrest.

The weaknesses of the model

Notwithstanding these apparently considerable strengths, post-war Marxism also contains fundamental analytic weaknesses. Its main weaknesses as a serious contender to the social democratic hegemony of most of the post-war period are threefold. The first weakness is rooted in the all-pervading determinism of the model. Although the model explicitly presents a theory of history and social change which understands the dynamic for social change to be social class struggle, the prospect of successful working class struggle is largely absent in the fine detail of the model. Historical and contemporary struggles between the two major social classes and between other social groups are seen implicitly, if not explicitly, as capable of resolution only by the victory of a dominant social class or group aided by the state.

As we have observed earlier, the struggle for citizen rights is seen as having elicited a response from the capitalist state aimed at, and largely successful in, incorporating all sections of the British population into the logic and values of capitalism (Saville, 1957; Mandel, 1968; Baran and Sweezy, 1968). Struggles for state welfare provision have resulted in similar outcomes. The capitalist state has utilised the struggles for state-provided health, education, income maintenance and other services to develop a welfare system which has functioned to satisfy the needs of capitalism rather than the needs of ordinary people. Social welfare interventions, whether in education, health or income maintenance provision are seen as having been determined, in large part, by the need to reinforce and recreate the norms and values of capitalist society. The provision of base-line income maintenance services and services in cash and kind are seen as part of a strategy of system maintenance and as a buffer against social unrest (see Chapter 4).

While this sort of approach has a kind of all-inclusive explanatory neatness about it, it poses problems on theoretical and empirical levels. In the first place, it is profoundly un-Marxist. It purports to be rooted in a set of social theories which have abstracted from the observation of social realities the lesson that progressive social change will occur as a result of the social and political struggles of a strong working class movement. None the less, in its detailed analysis of historical and contemporary struggles for welfare, it presents as rigid a puppet theatre model of state, society and social policy. The capitalist puppeteer (the state), acting on instructions from its employer (the ruling class), determines the outcome of each societal drama as surely as the beachside entertainer controls the outcome of each and every conflict between Punch and Judy. With the help of repressive or ideological state apparatuses (Althusser, 1971) – capitalist society's equivalent of the sometimes stern, sometimes caring policeman – the ruling class controls, or uses to its own advantage, the actions of the working class movement (Punch and Judy) even when those actions (political struggle) appear, as in each and every seaside performance, to be aimed at overthrowing the rule of law and the conventions of dominant society.

At an empirical level, the approach is equally unsatisfactory. The history of state welfare provision is marked by the selective opposition of large sections of industrial capitalism to state expenditure on welfare and by cacophonous complaints that welfare policies have failed, even if that were the intention to service the needs of capitalism. The empirical realities of post-war Britain, then, provide weak rather than strong foundations on which to build the Marxist functionalist edifice.

Other weaknesses are also evident in this critique of social democracy. On a theoretical level, it fails to give any satisfactory explanation of the claim that the state in capitalist society always acts to serve the interests of a capitalist class. On an empirical level, it appears to ignore any evidence which suggests that the state may have intervened in post-war civil society in ways which may not have reinforced or protected the interests of a capitalist class exclusively.

Finally, the fundamental basis of this perspective appears to be little more than a tautology. The state in post-war capitalist society is presented as a political directorate co-ordinating the interests of capitalism. Its main function is seen as the perpetuation of a capitalist system of social, economic and political organisation. The perpetuation of a capitalist system is seen as sufficient evidence of both the function of the state in capitalist societies and of its successful execution of that function. Consequently, all state activity is seen as necessarily determined, in intention and in outcome, by the state's *raison d'être* – the perpetuation of the capitalist system. Explanations of the durability of capitalism as a social and economic system which do not emphasise the pre-eminent role played by a ruling class through the mechanisms of the state, in maintaining that system are rarely considered and more rarely evaluated.

An increasingly strong body of evidence exists which indicates that an adequate understanding of the relationship between society, state and welfare must, while avoiding the rigid determinism of post-war Marxism, account for an apparent tendency for the state to act primarily in the interests of dominant or ruling sections of the population. Such an understanding would also need to suggest how, given such a relationship, some of the interests of a wide societal constituency may also be met, albeit secondarily and contingently, by the state.

More recently, this sort of attempt has been made by writers arguing within a left social democracy which has been influenced, but not swamped by post-war Marxism (Miliband, 1969, 1978, 1982; Poulantzas, 1972, 1975; Offe and Ronge, 1975; Ginsburg, 1979; Gough, 1979; Offe, 1984). This attempt to rehabilitate Marxism and social democracy suggests two important features of the modern capitalist state. First, that it is predisposed to act in the long-term interests of capitalism; but second, it possesses a degree of relative autonomy from ruling interests and has been particularly susceptible to change at times of heightened inter-class or intra-class struggle.

In order to come to some tentative conclusions about the strength of this attempt as a critique and explanatory model, we need to give some consideration to the evidence.

It has been argued that the conditions under which post-war state welfare developed supports the idea of a constrained but relatively autonomous state intervening in ways which demonstrate it to be acting in a tension between antagonistic and contradictory influences (Offe, 1984). As a consequence, the policies that emerge from the state are contradictory in their aims. Or so it is argued.

So how does this argument stand up to the empirical evidence? During this post-war period the British economy underwent an unprecedented expansion which led to both the depletion of labour reserves and to an increasingly strong labour movement. This period also saw an expansion in the range and functions of state intervention. There appears to be a *prima facie* case, at least, for an explanation that promotes the arguments that:

(a) during this period, interventionist policies were placed on the political agenda in response to labour movement pressure thus demonstrating a degree of relative autonomy for the state; and
(b) that the nature of the policies developed were, despite their provenance, deeply contradictory.

As we have seen earlier (Chapter 4), this might be seen to be reflected in policies on education, housing and income maintenance. Similarly, state social work, emerging out of the welfare state package, appears to have served contradictory functions during this period. An emphasis on rehabilitation rather than punishment quite clearly emerged in post-war social work (Packman, 1975; Jones, 1983). At the same time, however, an emphasis on ideas of family rather than structural pathology as the source of social ills (Jenkins, 1972; Joseph, 1972) placed social work practice equally clearly within the conformative apparatus of the state (Pearson, 1973; Corrigan and Leonard, 1978; Jones, 1983).

The changing focus of social work during the subsequent retrenchment of the economy in the 1970s and 1980s would also, on the face of it, point towards a model of understanding dependent on notions of relative autonomy and contradiction.

The establishment of unified social service departments in the early 1970s might well be seen as demonstrating both the relative autonomy of the state to act in the interests of a wide societal constituency and also the constraints within which that autonomy operated. In part, the Seebohm Committee's proposals reflected an acceptance of a structural pathology explanation of social problem causation. The 'rediscovery of poverty' school of thought appears to have convinced the committee that many of the problems social work confronted were socially rather than individually induced. The state, itself, acted to implement the universal departments which the committee saw as providing universalistic services but did so in a way (and with such resources) which limited the focus of intervention to the level of the family and served to entrench the notion of family pathology as the cause of social ills.

The development of community social work may also be seen as highlighting similar contradictions. State-sanctioned and financed community work may legitimately be seen as emerging as a strategy to integrate socially potentially alienated sections of British society. The decline of industry, especially in inner-city areas during the late 1960s, formed part of the restructuring of capitalism. It also appears to have precipitated a sense of alienation among those who lived in such areas who experienced, following the demise of indigenous industry, high levels of poverty, unemployment, housing problems and environmental blight. In such situations, the local and central state was perceived to have lost its legitimacy for at least certain sections of the population. The capitalist state, and indeed ruling interests, were therefore faced with a paradoxical problem. Capital accumulation must, perforce, be fostered but there was also a clear and urgent need to integrate socially a potentially malcontent inner-city working class. Community work was seen as the solution to this paradox (Bolger *et al.*, 1981; Loney, 1983). Community work was to function as a shock absorber to incorporate poor working class areas into mainstream society and to manage or mediate conflict between damaged communities and the local state (Gough, 1979). Community work projects, once established, were to operate within an ideology of community pathology and were to work to modify this pathology through facilitating community self-help. That this was the intention may well be demonstrated by the fate of radical Community Development Projects which developed a structural understanding of social problems (Loney, 1983). None the less, this example of welfare intervention can be seen as illustrating both the relative autonomy of the state and also the contradictory nature of welfare intervention.

That such projects and communities were resourced in the first place may well reflect the state's capacity to respond to perceived threat. That state-financed community work was expected to develop a community pathology-focused practice, aimed at social integration, may well demonstrate the limits of that autonomy. None the less, it may be argued that British community work in the 1970s and 1980s exposes the full limits of autonomy.

Contemporary community work represents much more than an ideological charade. In order for community work to function successfully in the interests of capitalism, it has perforce to develop real and direct relationships with working class people and communities. In doing so, it exposes a crucial contradiction which exists at the core of welfare provision: even interventions intended to control and integrate carry some potential for liberation. To develop direct relationships with the community in which they work, community workers introduce the possibility of participation and dialogue on community and wider issues. Policies and actions related to the long-term concerns of ruling interests have, on a number of issues from housing to employment, contained the promise – and sometimes the reality – of power through knowledge and participation (see Craig *et al.*, 1982; Loney, 1983).

Welfare intervention may have exposed a tension between the long-term interests of capitalism on the one hand and the interests of a wider constituency on the other.

Earlier post-war Marxism and the critical approach of the new left served both to expose the weaknesses of social democracy and, latterly, to rescue and reform it. Here the emphasis appeared to be on support for those state interventions which operated in the tension between the needs of capitalism and the needs of the polity. That tension and that attempt at rehabilitation were tackled head on by a radical right revival which started out from a position equally critical of the welfare state as that of the Marxists. This approach has had much more influence than the earlier Marxist critique in overshadowing social democracy's post-war welfare state.

Social democracy and the right: a critique and a refutation

In recent years the views of the radical right on welfare, as on other areas of state intervention, have become part of the currency of welfare, as well as political, debate. A perspective traditionally regarded with hostility by adherents to a wide range of views on the political spectrum, has been presented as the new political orthodoxy. The state provision of welfare and of much else has been characterised by the radical right as the source of many of Britain's social, economic and moral problems. The natural state of humankind is seen, from this perspective, as one in which individuals are free from regulation by the state (Hayek, 1980) and free to express natural individualism (Hayek, 1949).

Social democracy's welfare state has operated to limit individual freedom severely and also to place an economic burden on the British economy which ultimately led to a fiscal crisis.

With elegant rhetoric, the radical right offered an explanation of the failure of the British economy and the restructuring of welfare since the late 1960s. Social expenditure on welfare and other state activities in the post-war period had eaten up a growing proportion of gross national product. The non-productive sectors of the economy were, therefore, sapping the lifeblood of the productive sectors. The welfare state, in other words, had undermined the British economy. Such an analysis presents at least a *prima facie* case to be answered (see Bacon and Eltis, 1976, for an extended discussion of this issue).

Radical right views also emphasised the extent to which the provision of state welfare limits individual freedom to choose and also generates social cleavages. Authors from quite different political perspectives have argued that such views of state welfare are shared by the public at large (Klein, 1974; Harris and Seldon, 1979).

Only in a free market economy, argue the proponents of this approach, is freedom assured and social and economic ills remedied. This sort of approach is as problematic as the social democratic approach which it sought to replace

Implicit in Friedman's analysis of welfare as obliterating human freedom, for example, is the proposition that in the free market society, which the radical right poses in contradistinction to the welfare state society, freedom would be a natural concomitant of social and economic organisation. In doing so Friedman follows neo-classical economic theory which equates individual liberty with freedom. This must surely be a dubious equation because it ignores the effect that economic systems have on the distribution of power. The indisputable evidence to be drawn from the study of contemporary societies is that control of resources, especially of resources that are privately owned, gives resource-holders disproportionate power. Radical right economists and social theorists, like the neo-classical economists before them, ignore in their analysis that the freedom of the individual is contingent on the place that the individual occupies in the social structure.

As we have seen, another important plank in the radical right analysis and critique is that welfare is socially disruptive. It translates wants and needs into rights. It is unable to satisfy demand for those rights and thus creates social cleavages between would-be recipients of services. It would certainly appear that the general public regards some state services and benefits as directed inappropriately. Certainly, public attitudes to, say, the practice of income maintenance agencies supports the contentions of the radical right in this instance (Klein, 1974; Taylor-Gooby, 1985). It is, none the less, the case that surveys of public opinion demonstrate these contentions to be only partly sustainable. Recent evidence suggests that in respect of large areas of state provision (for example, in health and education) public attitudes support further taxation and thence social expenditure to secure wider rights of access to welfare services (Taylor-Gooby, 1985).

A further set of arguments marshalled by the radical right is concerned with the effect of welfare spending on the so-called productive sectors of the economy. Large scale state welfare provision, it is argued, reduces the incentive of entrepreneurial individuals to innovate. It is said to do so because, like all services provided as a result of public expenditure, it implies high levels of taxation and thus restricted levels of reward for the successful entrepreneur. Additionally, it is argued, welfare expenditure has no discernible positive impact on production. The former claim remains unsupported by any reliable evidence and there may, in fact, be evidence which strongly suggests that taxation does not reduce incentive to any great extent (Galbraith, 1963). The second argument is a little more difficult to despatch. Direct links between expenditure on welfare and wealth production are difficult to trace. However, consideration of the stated aims of certain social policies as aids to wealth creation may serve to cast some doubt on this particular anti-collectivist view.

A *prima facie* case can be constructed which offers strong suggestive evidence that social policies and welfare expenditure have, in fact, been used to create amenable conditions for increased industrial production and thence increased profit. Certainly, particular income maintenance and education policies introduced before the current economic recession would, at the very least, suggest that the industrial sector of the economy, as well as interventionist governments, perceived links between social expenditure and production and profit levels. One of the key pressure groups promoting the idea of a reorganisation of state secondary education in the late 1950s and the early 1960s was industrialists. A consistent complaint from the captains of British industry in the post-war period was that the then existing segregated system of secondary education acted as a brake on increased industrial production. It did so because that system failed to produce a reservoir of technologically competent industrial workers. A more flexible system of secondary education, such as that envisaged in the plans for comprehensivisation, was regarded by British industrialists as more likely to improve levels of production and profit in British industry (see Bellaby, 1977; Reynolds and Sullivan, 1987).

Similarly, income maintenance provisions including the original Beveridge proposals and the introduction, in 1966, of an earnings related unemployment benefit provide highly suggestive evidence of a perceived link between social intervention and expenditure on the one hand and production and profit on the other. The immediate post-war provisions, set in the context of technical, if not actual, full employment may be seen as having served two functions. In the first place, they provided an economic safety net to catch the frictionally unemployed and other minority groups. Secondarily, they provided a level of income for those whose earnings had been interrupted which maintained basic levels of consumption. Domestic levels of consumption, in an economy which had been severely damaged by the burdens of war, were not insignificantly associated with levels of production and profit.

The introduction of an earnings related unemployment benefit took place interestingly enough at a historical juncture when the

British economy was in the throes of an attempted move from labour intensive to capital intensive production. Government and state presented this social policy innovation as one which would help maintain the living standards of frictionally unemployed people. Evidence exists, however, which suggests that government, state and industry saw the new benefit as both placating those made unemployed by the restructuring of British industry and as maintaining domestic levels of consumption for more profitably produced products.

One final weakness of this approach relates to its implicit analysis of the relationship between state and government. Like the social democratic and industrial state perspectives, this perspective theorises the state as occupying a subservient or handmaiden position to government. Government, acting on a mandate from the population, makes policy, the organs of state execute that policy. Such a perspective would, therefore, suggest that governments pledged, like the Thatcher governments, to removing the state from substantial areas of interventionist activity in welfare might effect that intention more or less successfully. As we have seen in earlier chapters, the project of rolling back the state from substantial areas of welfare remains, despite the considerable restructuring of state activities, significantly incomplete (see also Taylor-Gooby, 1985). Whether this failure to determine state activity arises as a result of an under-estimation, in theory and action, of the degree of state power which has passed out of the hands of government in contemporary British society (Jessop, 1980; Cawson 1982), or results from other factors, it does indicate a marked weakness in the radical right perspective on state and welfare.

The radical right and modern social policy

Notwithstanding these weaknesses, the radical right has, as we have already seen, made its mark on modern social policy. Prime Ministers Thatcher and Major have, in creating a new social policy agenda, learnt the lessons of social democratic failure as well as contributing to its demise. This is clear in the extent to which both Premiers have created or maintained a party politicised senior civil service (Ingham, 1991; Sullivan, 1992). It is clear also in the way in which each has acknowledged and then countered a plurality of opinion in British society rather than assuming and fostering consensus. The growth of a British underclass during the 1980s and 1990s, if that is what it is, is an outcome of this approach. Its existence, growth and political insignificance is – perhaps more than anything else – proof of the death of old-style social democracy. Beveridge, as well as Keynes, now seems consigned to the political grave. For the political change is immense.

If post-war governments, formed by the Conservatives or by Labour, claimed political legitimacy, in part, from a moral, socially concerned consensus, then a turnaround appears to have occurred in the last fifteen years. Modern Conservatism appears to have maintained as well as created a complacent but dominant minority (consistently around 40 per cent of the electorate). The relative affluence and security, as well as the political loyalty of this group has had profound effects on social provision. For it acts as a strong counterbalance to a socially conscious but divided majority. In this situation and in protection of the minority's interests, social democracy's concern with the have-nots appears to have been buried by a culture of complacency (Galbraith, 1992).

This change in policy culture was in part created and is now in part sustained by the resurgence of a two-nation Conservatism. The premiership of Mrs Thatcher encouraged the growth in influence, and in some cases the formation, of proliferation of right-wing policy lobbies: the IEA, the Adam Smith Institute, the No Turning Back Group of right-wing Conservative MPs, the Social Affairs Unit, as well as the Centre for Policy Studies. These organisations, as well as having easier access to Conservative governments in the 1980s and 1990s than had been their experience in earlier post-war years, have attempted to underpin a revolution in thinking about social and economic policy. No small part in this process has been played by the steady stream of publications seeking to produce blueprints for a restructured welfare state. Though Conservative governments have ultimately balked at those prescriptions suggesting complete abolition, these groups have had more influence on the policy process than even the Fabian Society or the trades union movement exerted in periods of Labour government. Social policy in the 1990s has undergone a transformation compared with the earlier post-war period. The implications of this for future social policy are considered in detail elsewhere

(Glennerster and Midgley, 1991; Sullivan, 1992). Suffice it to say here that the present state of welfare and the partial, if not yet complete, reorientation of social policy can be interpreted in either of two ways.

First, and in my view most likely, the state of welfare in 1994 is a transitional stage between the old-style welfare state and a market welfare state based on managed or unmanaged competition. It is, at present, the enabling state. The question from this viewpoint is whether it is on the way to becoming the residual state. On this reading, any future non-Conservative government would find it difficult to turn back the clock, even if it wished to.

However, it might be possible to discern in government failure to eradicate the welfare state, comforting signs that governments in the 1990s will risk going no further than bolting the market onto welfare. Only time will tell.

Bibliography

Aaronovitch, S. (1981), *The Road from Thatcherism* (London: Lawrence & Wishart).

Aaronovitch, S. and Smith, R. (1981), *The Political Economy of British Capitalism* (London: McGraw-Hill).

Addison, P. (1982), *The Road to 1945* (London: Quartet).

Aitken, I. (1992), 'Raising a glass amid the doom', *The Guardian*, 13 April.

Allen, S. (ed.) (1974), *Conditions of Illusion* (London: Feminist Books).

Althusser, L. (1971), 'Ideology and ideological state apparatuses', in Althusser, L., *Lenin and Philosophy and Other Essays* (London: New Left Books).

Association of University Teachers (1989), *Annual Report* (London: Association of University Teachers).

Bacon, R. and Eltis, W. A. (1976), *Britain's Economic Problem: Too few producers* (London: Macmillan).

Bailey, J. (1980), *Ideas and Intervention: Social theory for practice* (London: Routledge & Kegan Paul).

Banks, O. (1981), *Faces of Feminism* (Oxford: Martin Robertson).

Baran, P. A. and Sweezy, P. M. (1968), *Monopoly Capital* (Harmondsworth: Penguin Books).

Barclay, P. (1982), *Social Workers: Their roles and tasks*, The Barclay Report. (London: Bedford Square Press).

Barker, J. (1979), 'Social conscience and social policy', *Journal of Social Policy*, vol. 8, no. 2, pp. 177–206.

Barker, R. (1978), *Political Ideas in Modern Britain* (London: Methuen).

Barnett, A. (1984), 'Beyond consensus', *New Socialist*, no. 18, pp. 33–5.

Barnett, S. (1896), *What Is Toynbee Hall?* (London: Toynbee Hall).

Barr, N., Glennerster, H. and LeGrand, J. (1988), *Reform and the National Health Service* (London: LSE).

Barratt-Brown, M. (1972), *From Labourism to Socialism* (Leeds: Spokesman Books).

Bean, P. and MacPherson, S. (eds) (1983), *Approaches to Welfare* (London: Routledge & Kegan Paul).

Bell, D. (1960), *The End of Ideology* (New York: Free Press).

Bellaby, P. (1977), *The Sociology of Comprehensive Schooling* (London: Methuen).

Benn, C. and Simon, B. (1972), *Half-Way There* (Harmondsworth: Penguin Books).

Benn, T. (1989), *Against the Tide* (London: Hutchinson).

Bessell, R. (1970), *Introduction to Social Work* (London: Batsford).

Bettelheim, B. (1969), *The Children of the Dream* (London: Thames & Hudson).

Beveridge, Sir W. (1942), *Social Insurance and Allied Services*, Cmnd 6404 (London: HMSO).

Blackburn, R. (1972), 'The new capitalism', in R. Blackburn (ed.) *Ideology in the Social Sciences* (London: Fontana).

Bolger, S., Corrigan, Paul, Docking, J. and Frost, N. (1981), *Towards Socialist Welfare Work* (London: Macmillan).

Bosanquet, N. (1983), *After the New Right* (London: Heinemann).

Bowlby, J. (1953), *Child Care and the Growth of Love* (Harmondsworth: Penguin Books).

Boyson, R. (ed.) (1971), *Down with the Poor* (London: Churchill Press).

Bremner, M. (1968), *Dependency and the Family* (London: Institute of Economic Affairs).

Bremner, R. (1974), 'Shifting attitudes', in P. E. Weinberger (ed.) *Perspectives on Social Welfare* (New York: Macmillan).

Brewer, C. and Lait, J. (1981) *Can Social Work Survive?* (London: Temple Smith).

Brittain, V. (1953), *Lady into Woman* (London: Dakers).

Bronfenbrenner, U. (1974), *Two Worlds of Childhood* (Harmondsworth: Penguin Books).

Brook, E. and Davis, A. (1985), *Women, the Family and Social Work* (London: Tavistock).

Brown, G. W. and Harris, T. (1978), *Social Origins of Depression* (London: Tavistock).

Brown, M. (1976), *Introduction to Social Administration* (London: Hutchinson).

Bruce, M. (1961), *The Coming of the Welfare State* (London: Batsford).

Calder, A. (1965), *The People's War* (London: Paladin).

Case Con Collective (1970), 'Case Con manifesto', *Case-Con, 1* (London: Case Con Collective).

Cawson, A. (1982), *Corporatism and Welfare* (London: Heinemann).

Chesler, P. (1972), *Women and Madness* (New York: Doubleday).

Chitty, C. (1989), *Towards a New Education System: The victory of the New Right?* (London: Falmer Press).

Clarke, J. (1980), 'Social democratic delinquents and Fabian families' in M. Fitzgerald (eds), *Permissiveness and Control* (London: Macmillan).

Coates, K. and Silburn, R. (1970), *Poverty, the Forgotten Englishman* (Harmondsworth: Penguin Books).

Coates, K. and Silburn, R. (1983), *Poverty, the Forgotten Englishman* 2nd edn (Leeds: Spokesman Books).

Cohen, S. (1975), 'It's alright for you to talk: political and sociological manifestos for social work action', in R. Bailey and M. Brake (eds), *Radical Social Work* (London: Edward Arnold).

Comer, L. (1971), *The Myth of Motherhood* (Leeds: Spokesman Pamphlets).

Conservative Party (1979), *Conservative Manifesto: 1979* (London: Conservative Central Office).

Conservative Party (1983), *Conservative Manifesto: 1983* (London: Conservative Central Office).

Conservative Party (1987), *Conservative Manifesto: 1987* (London: Conservative Central Office).

Corrigan, Paul (1975), 'Community work and political struggle', in P. Leonard (ed.) (1975), *The Sociology of Community Action* (Keele: University of Keele).

Corrigan, Paul (1977), 'The welfare state as an arena for class struggle', *Marxism Today* (March), pp. 87–93.

Corrigan, Paul (1979), 'Popular consciousness and social democracy', *Marxism Today* (December), pp. 14–17.

Corrigan, Paul and Leonard, P. (1978), *Social Work Practice under Capitalism* (London: Macmillan).

Corrigan, Philip (ed.) (1980), *Capitalism, State Formation and Marxist Theory* (London: Quartet).

Cowley, J., Kaye, A., Mayo, M. and Thompson, M. (eds) (1977), *Community or Class Struggle* (London: Stage One Publishing).

Cox, A. and Mead, M. (eds) (1975), *A Sociology of Medical Practice* (London: Collier-Macmillan).

Craig, G., Derricourt, N. and Loney, M. (eds) (1982), *Community Work and the State* (London: Routledge & Kegan Paul).

Crosland, C. A. R. (1952), 'The transition from capitalism', in R. H. S. Crossman (ed.), *New Fabian Essays* (London: Turnstile Press).

Crosland, C. A. R. (1956), *The Future of Socialism* (London: Jonathan Cape).

Crosland, C. A. R. (1974), *Socialism Now* (London: Jonathan Cape).

Crosland, S. (1982), *Tony Crosland* (London: Jonathan Cape).

Crossman, R. H. S. (1950), *Socialist Values in a Changing Society* (London: Fabian Society).

Crossman, R. H. S. (ed.) (1952), *New Fabian Essays* (London: Turnstile Press).

Crossman, R. H. S. (1975), *Diaries of a Cabinet Minister: Volume 1* (London: Jonathan Cape).

Curtis, M. (1946), *Report of the Committee on the Care of Children*, Cmnd 6922 (London: HMSO).

Dale, J. and Foster, P. (1986) *Feminists and State Welfare* (London: Routledge & Kegan Paul).

Dale, R. (1989) *The State and Education Policy* (London: Open University Press).

Dalton, K. (1969), *The Menstrual Cycle* (Harmondsworth: Penguin Books).

Dean, H. and Taylor-Gooby, P. (1991), *Dependency Culture* (Hemel Hempstead: Harvester Wheatsheaf).

Deem, R. (1978), *Women and Schooling* (London: Routledge & Kegan Paul).

Delamont, S. (1980) *Sex Roles and the School* (London: Methuen).

Department of Education and Science (1983), *Report of Her Majesty's Inspectors of Schools* (London: HMSO).

Department of Education and Science (1990), *Grant Maintained Schools* (London: DES).

Department of Health (1989), *Working for Patients* (London: HMSO).

Department of Health (1993), *NHS Trusts* (London: Department of Health).

Dicey, A. V. (1962), *Law and Public Opinion in England* (London: Macmillan) (1st edn published in 1914).

Donzelot, J. (1980), *The Policing of Families* (London: Hutchinson).

Doyal, L. (1983), *The Political Economy of Health* (London: Pluto Press).

Dunning, E. A., and Hopper, E. I. (1966), 'Industrialisation and the problem of convergence: a critical note', *Sociological Review*, vol. 14, no. 2, pp. 163–86).

Ehrenreich, B. and English, D. (1979), *For Her Own Good* (London: Pluto Press).

Elis Thomas, D. (1985), Unpublished paper delivered at British Association of Social Workers National Conference, University College of Swansea.

Enthoven, A. (1985), *Reflections on the Management of the NHS* (London: Nuffield Provincial Hospitals Trust).

Fenwick, I. G. K. (1976), *The Comprehensive School: 1940–1970* (London: Methuen).

Finch, J. and Groves, D. (eds) (1983), *Labour of Love* (London: Routledge & Kegan Paul).

Flatner, P. (1988), 'Education matters' in R. Jowell *et al.* (eds), *British Social Attitudes: The fifth report* (Aldershot: Gower).

Ford, J. (1969), *Social Class and the Comprehensive School* (London: Routledge & Kegan Paul).

Foot, M. (1975), *Aneurin Bevan: 1945–1960* (London: Paladin).

Forsyth, G. (1968), *Doctors and Medicine* (London: Pitman).

Friedman, M. (1962), *Capitalism and Freedom* (Chicago: Chicago University Press).

Friedman, M. and Friedman, R. (1980), *Free to Choose* (Harmondsworth: Penguin Books).

Furniss, N. and Tilton, T. (1979), *The Case for the Welfare State*, (Bloomington: Indiana University Press).

Galbraith, J. K. (1963), *American Capitalism* (Harmondsworth: Penguin Books).

Galbraith, J. K. (1972), *The New Industrial Society* (Harmondsworth: Penguin Books).

Galbraith, J. K. (1992), *The Culture of Contentment* (London: Sinclair-Stevenson).

Gamble, A. (1979), 'The decline of the Conservative Party', *Marxism Today* (November), pp. 6–12.

Gamble, A. (1980), 'Thatcher: make or break', *Marxism Today* (November), pp. 14–19.

Gamble, A. (1985), 'Smashing the state: Thatcher's radical crusade', *Marxism Today* (June), pp. 21–6.

Gamble, A. (1987), *The Free Economy and the Strong State* (London: Macmillan).

George, V. (1973), *Social Security and Society* (London: Routledge & Kegan Paul).

George, V. and Wilding, P. (1976), *Ideology and Social Welfare* (London: Routledge & Kegan Paul).

George, V. and Wilding, P. (1984), *The Impact of Social Policy* (London: Routledge & Kegan Paul).

George, V. and Wilding, P. (1985), *Ideology and Social Welfare* revised edn (London: Routledge & Kegan Paul).

Gieve, K. (1974), 'The independence demand', in S. Allen (ed.), *Conditions of Illusion* (London: Feminist Books).

Gilder, G. (1988), *Health and Poverty* (London: Buchan & Euright).

Ginsburg, N. (1979), *Class, Capital and Social Policy* (London: Macmillan).

Ginsburg, N. (1992), *Divisions of Welfare* (London: Sage).

Glazer, N. (1988), *The Limits of Social Policy* (Boston: Harvard University Press).

Glennerster, H. (1985), *Paying for Welfare*, (Oxford: Basil Blackwell).

Gold, D. A., Lo, C. Y. and Wright, E. O. (1975), 'Recent developments in Marxist theories of the state', *Monthly Review* (New York) vol. 27, no. 5.

Goldsmith, M. and Willetts, D. (1988), *Managed Health Care: A new system for a better service* (London: Centre for Policy Studies).

Goldthorpe, J. H. (1962), 'The development of Social Policy in England', *Transactions of the 5th World Congress of Sociology.*

Gough, I. (1975), 'State expenditure in advanced capitalism', *New Left Review*, vol. 92, pp. 53–92.

Gough, I. (1979), *The Political Economy of the Welfare State* (London: Macmillan).

Gove, W. R., and Tudor, J. F. (1973), 'Adult sex roles and mental illness', *American Journal of Sociology*, vol. 78, pp. 812–35.

Green, D. (1982), *The New Right* (London: Macmillan).

Greenleaf, W. H. (1983), *The British Political Tradition: The rise of collectivism* (London: Methuen).

Greenleaf, W. H. (1987), *The British Political Tradition: A much governed nation* (London: Methuen).

Gregg, P. (1967), *The Welfare State: An economic and social history of Great Britain from 1945 to the present day* (London: Harrap).

Griffith, B., Iliffe, S. and Rayner, G. (1987), *Banking on Sickness: Commercial medicine in Britain and the USA* (London: Lawrence & Wishart).

Griffiths, B. (1983), *The Moral Basis of the Market Economy* (London: Conservative Political Centre).

Griffiths, R. (1983), *NHS Management Enquiry* (London: HMSO).

Gulbenkian Foundation (1968), *Community Work and Social Change* (London: Longmans).

Habermas, J. (1976), *Legitimation Crisis* (London: Heinemann).

Hadley, R. and Cooper, M. (1984), *Patch-based Social Services Teams* (Lancaster: Department of Social Administration, University of Lancaster).

Hadley, R., Cooper, M., Dale, P. and Stacy, G. (1987), *A Community Social Worker's Handbook* (London: Tavistock).

Hadley, R., Dale, P. and Sills, P. (1984), *Decentralising Social Services: A model for change* (London: Bedford Square Press).

Hall, Penelope (1952), *The Social Services of Modern England* (London: Routledge & Kegan Paul).

Hall, Phoebe, Land, H., Parker, R. and Webb, A. (1978), *Change, Choice and Conflict in Social Policy* (London: Heinemann).

Hall, S. (1979), 'The great moving right show', *Marxism Today* (January), pp. 14–20.

Hall, S. (1988), *The Hard Road to Renewal*, (London: Verso).

Hall, S., Critcher, C., Jefferson, T., Clarke, J. and Roberts, B. (1979), *Policing the Crisis* (London: Macmillan).

Hall, S. and Jacques, M. (1985). *The Politics of Thatcherism* (London: Lawrence & Wishart).

Halmos, P. (1965), *The Faith of the Counsellors* (London: Constable).

Halmos, P. (1978), *The Personal and the Political* (London: Hutchinson).

Halsey, A. H., Heath, A. F. and Ridge, J. M. (1980), *Origins and Destinations* (Oxford: Oxford University Press).

Ham, C. (1992), *The New National Health Service* (Oxford: Radcliffe Medical Press).

Handler, J. (1973), *The Coercive Social Worker* (Chicago: Rand McNally).

Harrington, W. and Young, P. (1978), *The 1945 Revolution* (London: Davis-Poynter).

Harris, D. (1987), *Justifying State Welfare* (Oxford, Basil Blackwell).

Harris, L. (1984), 'State and economy in the Second World War', in G. McLennan, D. Held and S. Hall (eds), *State and Society in Contemporary Britain* (Cambridge: Polity Press).

Harris, R. (1972), *Choice in Welfare* (London: Institute of Economic Affairs).

Harris, R. and Seldon, A. (1979), *Overruled on Welfare* (London: Institute of Economic Affairs).

Harris, R. and Seldon, A. (1987), *Welfare Without the State* (London: Institute of Economic Affairs).

Harrison, R. (1965), *Before the Socialists* (London: Routledge & Kegan Paul).

Hart, J. T. (1975), 'The inverse care law', in A. Cox and M. Mead (eds), *A Sociology of Medical Practice* (London: Collier-Macmillan).

Hartman, H. (ed.) (1981), *The Unhappy Marriage of Marxism and Feminism* (London: Pluto Press).

Hattersley, R. (1989), 'Afterword', in K. Hoover and R. Plant (eds), *Conservative Capitalism* (London: Routledge and Kegan Paul).

Hayek, F. A. (1944), *The Road to Serfdom* (London: Routledge & Kegan Paul).

Hayek, F. A. (1949), *Individualism and the Economic Order* (London: Routledge & Kegan Paul).

Hayek, F. A. (1960), *The Constitution of Liberty* (London: Routledge & Kegan Paul).

Hayek, F. A. (1973), *Law, Legislation and Liberty* Vol. 1 (London: Routledge & Kegan Paul).

Hayek, F. A. (1976), *Law, Legislation and Liberty* Vol. 2 (London: Routledge & Kegan Paul).

Hayek, F. A. (1979), *Law, Legislation and Liberty* Vol. 3 (London: Routledge & Kegan Paul).

Hayek, F. A. (1980), *1980s Unemployment and the Unions* (London: Institute of Economic Affairs).

Held, D. (ed.) (1982), *Classes, Power and Conflict* (London: Macmillan).

Held, D. and Hall, S. (eds) (1983), *States and Societies* (Oxford: Martin Robertson).

Hennessy, P. (1992), *Never Again* (London: Jonathan Cape).

Heraud, B. (1970), *Sociology and Social Work* (Oxford: Pergamon Press).

Hill, M. (1990) *Social Security Policy in Britain* (Aldershot: Edward Elgar).

Hill, M. (1993), *The Welfare State in Britain: A political history since 1945* (Aldershot: Edward Elgar).

Hills, J. (1990), *The State of Welfare* (Oxford: Clarendon Press).

Higgins, J. (1988), *The Business of Medicine* (London: Macmillan).

Higgins, J. (1990), *Caring for People, the Government's Proposal for Community Care* (Southampton: Institute of Health Policy Studies).

Hobsbawm, E. (1964), *Labouring Men* (London: Weidenfeld & Nicholson).

Hollingshead, A. and Redlich, R. C. (1958), *Social Class and Mental Illness* (New York: John Wiley).

Holman, R. (1978), *Poverty: Explanations of social deprivation* (Oxford: Martin Robertson).

Home Office (1965), *The Child, the Family and the Young Offender* Cmnd 2742 (London: HMSO).

Home Office (1968), *Children in Trouble* Cmnd 3601 (London: HMSO).

Howe, Sir G. (1983), 'Agenda for liberal Conservatism', *Journal of Economic Affairs* (January).

Ingham, B. (1991), *Kill the Messenger* (London: Harper Collins).

Jenkins, Roy (1972), *What Matters now* (London: Fontana).

Jessop, Bob (1977), 'Recent theories of the capitalist state', *Cambridge Journal of Economics*, vol. 1, pp. 353–73.

Jessop, B. (1980), 'The transformation of the state in post-war Britain', in R. Scase (ed.), *The State in Western Europe* (London: Croom Helm).

Johnson, N. (1991), *Restructuring the Welfare State* (Hemel Hempstead: Harvester Wheatsheaf).

Jones, Chris (1983), *State Social Work and the Working Class* (London: Macmillan).

Jones, H. (1971), *Crime in a Changing Society* (Harmondsworth: Penguin Books).

Jones, H. (ed.) (1981), *Society against Crime* (Harmondsworth: Penguin Books).

Jones, K. (1991), *The Making of Social Policy in Britain: 1830–1990* (London: The Athlone Press).

Jordan, B. (1974), *Poor Parents* (London: Routledge & Kegan Paul).

Jordan, B. (1981), *Automatic Poverty* (London: Routledge & Kegan Paul).

Joseph, Sir K. (1972), 'The cycle of deprivation', speech delivered to a conference of the Pre-school Play Association, 29 June.

Joseph, Sir K. (1976), *Stranded on the Middle Ground* (London: Centre for Policy Studies).

Joseph, Sir K. and Sumption, J. (1979), *Equality* (London: John Murray).

Jowell, R., Witherspoon, S. and Brook, L. (1989), *British Social Attitudes: The sixth report* (Aldershot: Gower).

Jowell, R., Witherspoon, S. and Brook, L. (1990) *British Social Attitudes: The seventh report* (Aldershot: Gower).

Jowell, R., Witherspoon, S. and Brook, L. (1991), *British Social Attitudes: The eighth report* (Aldershot: Gower).

Katz, M. (1989), *In the Shadow of the Poorhouse* (New York: Basic Books).

Kerr, C., Dunlop, J. T., Harbison, F. H. and Myers, C. A. (1962), *Industrialism and Industrial Man* (London: Heinemann).

Kincaid, J. (1973), *Poverty and Equality in Britain* (Harmondsworth: Penguin Books).

Kinnock, N. (1985), *The Future of Socialism* (London: Fabian Society).

Kinnock, N. (1991), 'Labour social policies', *Community Care*, 6 and 13 June.

Klein, R. (1974), *Social Policy and Public Expenditure* (London: Centre for Studies in Social Policy).

Klein, R. (1983), *The Politics of the N.H.S.* (Oxford: Blackwell).

Kogan, M. (1971), *The Politics of Education* (Harmondsworth: Penguin Books).

Kuenstler, P. (1961), *Community Organisation in Great Britain* (London: Faber).

Labour Party (1964), *Let's Go with Labour for the New Britain* (London: Labour Party).

Labour Party (1987), *Manifesto* (London: Labour Policy).

Labour Party (1989), *Policy Review Document on Local Government* (London: Labour Party).

Labour Party (1990), *Policy Review Document on Health* (London: Labour Party).

Labour Party (1991), *A Fresh Start for Health* (London: Labour Party).

Labour Party Research Department (1985), *Breaking the Nation* (London: Pluto Press/New Socialist).

Lafitte, F. (1962), *Social Policy in a Free Society* (Birmingham: University of Birmingham).

Land, H. (1978), 'Who cares for the family?', *Journal of Social policy*, vol. 7, pp. 257–84).

Laski, H. J. (1934), *The State in Theory and Practice* (London: Allen & Unwin).

Lawson, N. (1981), *The New Conservatism* (London: Conservative Political Centre).

Lawson, R. and Wilson, W. (1990), Poverty, Inequality and the Crisis of Social Policy (Washington, D.C.: Joint Center for Political and Economic Studies).

Leathard, A. (1991), *Health Care Provision: Past, present and future* (London: Chapman Hall).

Lees, D. (1961), *Health through Choice* (London: Institute of Economic Affairs).

Leeson, J. and Gray, J. (1978), *Women and Medicine* (London: Tavistock).

LeGrand, J. (1982), *The Strategy of Equality* (London: Allen & Unwin).

LeGrand, J. and Robinson, R. (eds) (1984), *Privatisation and the Welfare State* (London: Allen & Unwin).

Lejeune, A. (ed.) (1970), *Enoch Powell* (London: Stacey).

Leonard, P. (1975), 'Towards a paradigm for radical practice', in R. Bailey and M. Brake (eds), *Radical Social Work* (London: Edward Arnold).

Leonard P. (1979), 'Restructuring the welfare state', *Marxism Today* (December), pp. 7–13.

Leonard, P. (1983), 'Marxism, the individual and the welfare state', in P. Bean and S. MacPherson (eds), *Approaches to Welfare* (London: Routledge & Kegan Paul).

Lewis, J. (1973), 'Beyond suffrage: English feminism in the 1920s', *The Maryland Historian*, no. 6, pp. 1–17.

Lewis, O. (1961), *The Children of Sanchez* (New York: Random House).

Lidbetter, E. J. (1933), *Heredity and the Social Problem Group* (London: Edward Arnold).

London Edinburgh Weekend Return Group (1980), *In and against the State* (London: Pluto Press).

Loney, M. (1983), *Community against Government* (London: Heinemann).

Loney, M., Boswell, D. and Clarke, J. (1984), *Social Policy and Social Welfare* (Milton Keynes: Open University Press).

Longford, F. (1966), *Crime: A challenge to us all* (London: Labour Party).

McIntosh, M. (1984), 'The family, regulation and the public sphere', in G. McLennan, D. Held and S. Hall (eds), *State and Society in Contemporary Britain* (Cambridge: Polity Press).

Mack, J. and Lansley, S. (1985), *Poor Britain* (London: Allen & Unwin).

McLennan, G., Held, D. and Hall, S. (eds) (1983), *States and Societies* (Cambridge: Polity Press).

McLennan, G., Held, D. and Hall, S. (1984), *The Idea of the Modern State* (Milton Keynes: Open University Press).

McLeod, I. and Powell, J. E. (1952), *The Social Services* (London: Conservative Political Centre).

Mandel, E. (1968), *Marxist Economic Theory* (London: Merlin).

Marquand, D. (1992),'Major returns to bury Thatcherism, not praise it', *The Guardian*, 18 April.

Marshall, T. H. (1963), 'Citizenship and social class', in Marshall, T. H. (ed.), *Sociology at the Crossroads* (London: Heinemann).

Marshall, T. H. (1965), *Social Policy* (London: Hutchinson).

Marshall, T. H. (1971), 'Value problems of welfare capitalism', *Journal of Social Policy*, vol. 1, no. 1.

Marshall, T. H. (1975), *Social Policy* revised edn (London: Hutchinson).

Martin, A. (1913), 'The mother and social reform', in *Married Women and Social Reform*, in the journal *Nineteenth Century*.

Marwick, A. (1974), *War and Social Change in the Twentieth Century* (London: Macmillan).

Marwick, A. (1980), *Class, Image and Reality in Britain, France and the USA since 1930* (London: Collins).

Marwick, A. (1982), *British Society since 1945* (Harmondsworth: Penguin Books).

Marx, K. (1967), *Capital* (London: Dent).

Marx, K. (1973), 'The Eighteenth Brumaire of Louis Bonaparte', in D. Fernbach (ed.), *Marx: Surveys from exile* (Harmondsworth: Penguin Books).

Marx, K. and Engels, F. (1967), *The Communist Manifesto* (Harmondsworth: Penguin Books).

Maude, A. (1977), *The Right Approach to the Economy* (London: Conservative Political Centre).

Meyer, P. (1983), *The Child and the State* (Cambridge: CUP).

Middlemas, K. (1979), *Politics in Industrial Society* (London: André Deutsch).

Miliband, R. (1969), *The State in Capitalist Society* (London: Weidenfeld & Nicholson).

Miliband, R. (1978), *Marxism and Politics* (Oxford: OUP).

Miliband, R. (1982), *Capitalist Democracy in Britain* (Oxford: OUP).

Mills, C. Wright (1943), 'The professional ideology of social pathologists', *American Journal of Sociology*, vol. 49.

Mills, C. Wright (1959), *The Sociological Imagination* (Oxford: OUP).

Minford, P. (1983), *Unemployment: Cause and cure* (Oxford: Martin Robertson).

Minford, P. (1984), 'State expenditure: a study in waste', *Economic Affairs* May/June.

Mishra, R. (1975), 'Marx and welfare', *Sociological Review*, vol. 23, no. 2, pp. 287–313.

Mishra, R. (1981), *Society and Social Policy* (London: Macmillan).

Mishra, R. (1984), *The Welfare State in Crisis* (Brighton: Wheatsheaf).

Mishra, R. (1990), *The Welfare State in Capitalist Society* (Hemel Hempstead: Harvester Wheatsheaf).

Morgan, K. O. (1990), *The People's Peace* (London: OUP).

Mount, F. (1982), *The Subversive Family* (London: Jonathan Cape).

Munday, B. (1972), 'What is happening to social work students?', *Social Work Today*, Vol. 3, no. 6.

Murray, C. (1984), *Losing Ground* (New York: Basic Books).

Murray, C. (1990), *The Emerging British Underclass* (London: Institute for Economic Affairs).

National Advisory Board for Higher Education (1984), *Report* (London: NAB).

National Institute for Economic and Social Research (1991), *Economic Review* (136) (London: NIESR).

Novarra, V. (1980), *Women's Work, Men's Work: The ambivalence of equality* (London: Boyars).

No Turning Back Group (1988), *The NHS: A suitable case for treatment* (London: Conservative Political Centre).

NSPCC (1984), 'An overview of the research on the effects of unemployment on the family with particular reference to child abuse', *Information Briefing* no. 1 (London: NSPCC).

Oakley, A. (1974), *The Sociology of Housework* (Oxford: Martin Robertson).

O'Connor, J. (1973), *The Fiscal Crisis of the State* (New York: St Martin's Press).

O'Connor, J. (1984), *Accumulation Crisis* (New York: St Martin's Press).

Offe, C. (1982), 'Some contradictions of the modern welfare state', *Critical Social Policy*, vol. 2, no. 2, pp. 7–16.

Offe, C. (1984), *Contradictions of the Welfare State* (London: Hutchinson).

Offe, C. and Ronge, V. (1975), 'Theses on the theory of the state', *New German Critique*, vol. 6, pp. 139–47.

O'Higgins, M. (1983a), 'Rolling back the welfare state', in C. Jones and J. Stevenson (eds), Yearbook of Social Policy, 1982 (London: Routledge & Kegan Paul).

O'Higgins, M. (1983b), 'Inequality, redistribution and recession: the British Experience 1976–1982', *Journal of Social Policy* vol. 14, no. 3.

Olsen, M. R. (ed.) (1984), *Social Work and Mental Health* (London: Tavistock).

Packman, J. (1975), *The Child's Generation* (Oxford: Blackwell and Martin Robertson).

Papadakis, E. and Taylor-Gooby, P. (1987) *The Private Provision of Public Welfare* (Hemel Hempstead: Harvester Wheatsheaf).

Parker, J. (1975), *Social Policy and Citizenship* (London: Macmillan).

Parkinson, M. (1970), *The Labour Party and the Organisation of Secondary Education 1918–65* (London: Routledge & Kegan Paul).

Parry, N., Rustin, M. and Satyamurti, C. (eds) (1979), *Social Work, Welfare and the State* (London: Edward Arnold).

Parton, N. and Thomas, T. (1983), 'Child abuse and citizenship', in B. Jordan and N. Parton (eds), *The Political Dimensions of Social Work* (Oxford: Blackwell).

Pascall, G. (1983), 'Women and social welfare', in P. Bean and S. MacPherson (eds), *Approaches to Welfare* (London: Routledge & Kegan Paul).

Paton, C. (1991), *Competition and Planning in the NHS; the Danger of Unplanned Markets* (London: Chapman Hall).

Pearce, F. (1973), 'The British road to incorporation', *The Writing on the Wall*, vol. 2.

Pearson, G. (1973), 'Social work as the privatised solution to public ills', *British Journal of Social Work*, vol. 3, no. 2, pp. 209–23.

Philp, A. F. (1963), *Family Failure* (London: Faber).

Pimlott, B. (1988), 'The myth of consensus', in L. Smith (ed.), *The Making of Britain: Echoes of greatness* (London: Macmillan).

Pimlott, B. (1992), Harold Wildon (London: Harper Collins).

Pirie, M. and Butler E. (1988), *The Health of Nations* (London: Adam Smith Institute).

Plant, R. and Barry, N. (1990), *Citizenship and Rights in Thatcher's Britain* (London: Institute for Economic Affairs).

Poulantzas, N. (1972), 'The problem of the capitalist state', in R. Blackburn (ed.), *Ideology in the Social Sciences* (London: Fontana).

Poulantzas, N. (1973), *Political Power and Social Classes* (London: New Left Books).

Poulantzas, N. (1975), *Classes in Contemporary Society* (London: New Left Books).

Powell, J. E. (1966), *Medicine and Politics* (London: Pitman).

Powell, J. E. (1969), *Freedom and Reality* (London: Elliot Rightway Books).

Powell, J. E. (1972), *Still to Decide* (London: Elliot Rightway Books).

Rapoport, R., Rapoport, N. and Strelitz, Z. (1977), *Fathers, Mothers and Others* (London: Routledge & Kegan Paul).

Redwood, J. and Hatch, J. (1982), *Controlling Public Industries* (Oxford: Blackwell).

Reynolds, D. and Sullivan, M. (1987), *The Comprehensive Experiment* (Brighton: Falmer Press).

Riddell, P. (1983), *The Thatcher Government* (Oxford: Martin Robertson).

Robbins, Lord (1963), *Report on Higher Education*, Cmnd 2514 (London: HMSO).

Robertson, D. J., and Hunter, L. C. (1970), *Labour Market Issues of the 1970s* (Edinburgh: Oliver & Boyd).

Robertson, J. (1962), *Hospitals and Children* (London: Gollancz).

Robson, W. (1976), *Welfare State and Welfare Society* (London: Allen & Unwin).

Rodgers, B. (1969), *The Battle Against Poverty* (London: Routledge & Kegan Paul).

Roof, M. (1972), *A Hundred Years of Family Welfare* (London: Michael Joseph).

Rowthorn, B. (1981), 'The politics of the alternative economic strategy', *Marxism Today*, January.

Rubinstein, D. and Simon, B. (1973), *The Evolution of the Comprehensive School 1926–1972* (London: Routledge & Kegan Paul).

Rutter, M. (1975), *Maternal Deprivation Reassessed* (Harmondsworth: Penguin Books).

Rutter, M., and Madge, N. (1977), *Cycles of Disadvantage* (London: Heinemann).

Ryan, W. (1971), *Blaming the Victim* (New York: Random House).

Sainsbury, E. (1977), *The Personal Social Services* (London: Pitman).

Saville, J. (1957), 'The welfare state: an historical approach', *New Reasoner*, vol. 3.

Scase, R. (ed.) (1980), *The State in Western Europe* (London: Croom Helm).

Schott, K. (1984), 'The use of Keynesian economics: Britain 1940–64', *Economy and Society*, vol. 11, no. 3 (reproduced in G. McLennan,

D. Held and S. Hall (eds), *State and Society in Contemporary Britain* (Cambridge: Polity Press)).

Seebohm, Sir F. (1968), *Report of the Committee on Local Authority and Allied Personal Social Services*, Cmnd 3703 (London: HMSO).

Seed, P. (1973), *The Expansion of Social Work in Britain* (London: Routledge & Kegan Paul).

Seldon, A. (1967), *Taxation and Welfare* (London: Institute of Economic Affairs).

Seldon, A. (1977), *Charge* (London: Temple Smith).

Seldon, A. (1981), *Wither the Welfare State* (London: Institute of Economic Affairs).

Seldon, A. (1986), *The Riddle of the Voucher* (London: Institute of Economic Affairs).

Simon, B. (1988), *Bending the Rules* (London: Lawrence & Wishart).

Sked, A. and Cook, C. (1979), *Post War Britain: A political history* (Harmondsworth: Penguin Books).

Slack, K. (1966), *Social Administration and the Citizen* (London: Michael Joseph).

Steadman Jones, G. (1971), *Outcast London* (Oxford: OUP).

Sullivan, M. (1984), 'The crisis in welfare?', unpublished paper presented to School of Social Studies Colloquium, University College of Swansea.

Sullivan, M. (1987), *Sociology and Social Welfare* (London: Allen and Unwin).

Sullivan, M. (1989), *The Social Politics of Thatcherism: New Conservatism and the welfare state* (Swansea: University of Wales).

Sullivan, M. (1990), 'Communities and Social Policy', in Jenkins, R. and Edwards, A. (eds), *Towards the Year 2000* (Llandysul: Gower).

Sullivan, M. (1991), *The Labour Party and Social Reform* (Cardiff: University of Wales).

Sullivan, M. (1992), *The Politics of Social Policy* (Hemel Hempstead: Harvester Wheatsheaf).

Sullivan, M. (1994), *Labour and Social Reform: Social policy-making in a political party* (London: Merlin Press).

Tawney, R. H. (1964), *The Radical Tradition* (Harmondsworth: Penguin Books).

Taylor-Gooby, P. (1985), *Public Opinion, Ideology and State Welfare* (London: Routledge & Kegan Paul).

Taylor-Gooby, P. (1991), *Social Change, Social Welfare and Social Science* (Hemel Hempstead: Harvester Wheatsheaf).

Taylor-Gooby, P. and Dale, J. (1981), *Social Theory and Social Welfare* (London: Edward Arnold).

Thatcher, M. (1977), *Let Our Children Grow Tall* (London: Centre for Policy Studies).

Thompson, E. P. (1963), *The Making of the English Working Class* (London: Gollancz).

Thompson, G. (1984), 'Rolling back the state: economic intervention 1975–82', in G. McLennan, D. Held, and S. Hall (eds), *State and Society in Contemporary Britain* (Cambridge: Polity Press).

Timms, N. (1967), *Psychiatric Social Work in Great Britain* (London: Routledge & Kegan Paul).

Timms, N. and Watson, D. (eds) (1976), *Talking about Welfare* (London: Routledge & Kegan Paul).

Titmuss, R. (1963), *Essays on the Welfare State* (London: Allen & Unwin).

Townsend, P. (1974), 'The cycle of deprivation: the history of a confused thesis', in J. Thomas (ed.), *The Cycle of Deprivation* (Birmingham: BASW Publications).

Townsend, P. (1979) *Poverty in the UK* (Harmondsworth: Penguin).

Townsend P. and Abel-Smith, B. (1965), *The Poor and the Poorest* (London: Bell).

Townsend, P. and Davidson, N. (1982), *Inequalities in Health* (Harmondsworth: Penguin Books).

University Grants Committee (1984), *Strategy Document* (London: UGC).

Valentine, C. A. (1968), *Culture and Poverty* (Chicago: Chicago University Press).

Walker, A. (1983), 'Conservative social policy: the economic consequences', in Bull, D. and Wilding, P. (eds), Thatcherism and the Poor (London: CPAG).

Walker, A. and Walker, C. (1987), *The Growing Divide* (London: CPAG).

Walton, R. (1975), *Women in Social Work* (London: Routledge & Kegan Paul).

Whetham, W. C. D. (1909), *The Family and the Nation* (London: Longman and Green).

Wilensky, H. L. and Lebaux, C. N. (1965), *Industrial Society and Social Welfare* (New York: Free Press).

Willcocks, A. (1967), *The Creation of the National Health Service* (London: Routledge & Kegan Paul).

Williams, F. (1969), 'A Prime Minister remembers', in A. King (ed.), *The British Prime Minister* (London: Macmillan).

Williams, Fiona (1991) *Social Policy: A critical introduction* (Cambridge: Polity Press).

Williams, G. A. (1968), *Artisans and Sans Culottes* (London: Edward Arnold).

Williams, S. (1981), *Politics Is for People* (Harmondsworth: Penguin Books).

Williamson, B. (1990), *Temper of the Times* (Oxford: Blackwell).

Wilson, E. (1977), *Women and the Welfare State* (London: Tavistock).

Wilson, E. (1980), 'Feminism and social work', in M. Brake and R. Bailey (eds) *Radical Social Work and Practice* (London: Edward Arnold).

Wilson, E. (1981), *Only Half Way to Paradise* (London: Tavistock).

Wilson, H. and Herbert, G. (1978), *Parenting in the Inner City* (London: Routledge & Kegan Paul).

Woodroofe, K. (1971), *From Charity to Social Work* (London: Routledge & Kegan Paul).

Wooton, B. (1959), *Social Science and Social Pathology* (London: Allen & Unwin).

Young, H. (1989), *One of Us* (London: Macmillan).

Index